Techniques in
Complete
Denture Technology

Techniques in Complete Denture Technology

Tony Johnson
PhD, MMedSci, LCGI, MCGI, FETC, FHEA
Senior Lecturer
Academic Unit of Restorative Dentistry
School of Clinical Dentistry
University of Sheffield
UK

Duncan J. Wood
BMedSci, PhD, FHEA
Senior University Teacher
Academic Unit of Restorative Dentistry
School of Clinical Dentistry
University of Sheffield
UK

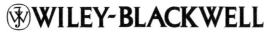

WILEY-BLACKWELL

A John Wiley & Sons, Ltd., Publication

This edition first published 2012
© 2012 by Tony Johnson and Duncan J. Wood

Wiley-Blackwell is an imprint of John Wiley & Sons, formed by the merger of Wiley's global
Scientific, Technical and Medical business with Blackwell Publishing.

Registered office: John Wiley & Sons, Ltd, The Atrium, Southern Gate, Chichester, West
                        Sussex, PO19 8SQ, UK

Editorial offices: 9600 Garsington Road, Oxford, OX4 2DQ, UK
                        The Atrium, Southern Gate, Chichester, West Sussex, PO19 8SQ, UK
                        2121 State Avenue, Ames, Iowa 50014-8300, USA

For details of our global editorial offices, for customer services and for information about
how to apply for permission to reuse the copyright material in this book please see our
website at www.wiley.com/wiley-blackwell.

Library of Congress Cataloging-in-Publication Data
Johnson, Tony (Anthony Phillip)
   Techniques in complete denture technology / Tony Johnson, Duncan J. Wood.
      p. ; cm.
   Includes bibliographical references and index.
   ISBN 978-1-4051-7909-6 (pbk. : alk. paper)
   I. Wood, Duncan J.   II. Title.
   [DNLM: 1. Denture, Complete.   2. Technology, Dental–methods.   WU 530]
   617.6'92–dc23

                                                        2011042661

A catalogue record for this book is available from the British Library.

Wiley also publishes its books in a variety of electronic formats. Some content that appears
in print may not be available in electronic books.

Set in 10/12 pt Calibri by Toppan Best-set Premedia Limited, Hong Kong

1   2012

Contents

As the dental profession becomes more successful in delaying complete edentulism in patients until much later in their lives, it also brings with it greater problems in providing these older patients with satisfactory complete dentures. More understanding of all aspects of complete denture provision will be needed to achieve satisfactory outcomes for these patients.

The technical aspects of complete denture provision are very often given brief consideration in publications relating to complete denture provision. This side of complete denture provision, however, often has a major impact on the success or failure of the dentures.

This book is intended for all student dentists and technicians, clinicians, clinical dental technicians and technicians who have an interest in complete denture provision, with the hope that it may stimulate new ideas and improve technique when considering the technical aspects of denture construction.

We would like to thank the following people who either provided or modelled for the pictures that appear in this text. First we thank Mr Peter Bridgwood for kindly allowing the use of his image and Dr Hannah Barnes for providing clinical pictures. We also appreciate the help given by David Wildgoose, Eleanor Stone, Laura Peacock, Sebastian Wilkins, Micheal Spencer, Daniel Leung, Lisa Smith, Christopher Povey and Anna Burrows.

Tony Johnson
Duncan Wood

Chapter 1 INTRODUCTION

This text will set out the ideal properties of complete dentures, and provide you with techniques for achieving these when carrying out any stage in the production process. Dentures should function well and look good. The denture wearer may value function over aesthetics or vice versa, but failure to establish a minimal requisite will lead to disappointment.

What do we mean by function well? Dentures should be comfortable, retentive, stable when biting together in any position, and restore the speech.

What do we mean by look good? Dentures should replace the teeth and the resorbed bone, resulting in natural looking anterior teeth, support of the soft tissues and restoration of any loss in vertical dimension.

Establishing function and aesthetics may be challenging in some cases, this text aims to provide the solutions to ensure the reader understands and can provide the various elements that are essential for optimum denture provision. This text will help the reader evaluate, design and provide the following requirements.

Fit: This is a result of impression technique, impression materials, model materials, processing method, denture base material and final fitting.

Retention: This results from fit and forming a border seal. Providing retention may prove difficult for lower dentures where stability and muscular control must be optimised to compensate.

Stability is dependent upon fit and occlusion. Establishing a balanced occlusion is key to maintaining stability and in turn the border seal. Lower dentures are particularly vulnerable to instability as a result of poor retention. Here the occlusal table should be designed to provide optimum load distribution in order to seat the denture.

Occlusion of the denture teeth may be established as a conventional balanced occlusion or as a lingualised scheme, each should result in multiple tooth contacts around the denture, providing stability in any position.

Muscular control provides long-term retention of the denture and is aided by the positioning of the teeth in the neutral zone and by the considered shaping of the polished surfaces of the denture.

Techniques in Complete Denture Technology, First Edition. Tony Johnson, Duncan J. Wood.
© 2012 Tony Johnson and Duncan J. Wood. Published 2012 by Blackwell Publishing Ltd.

Aesthetics of dentures are undoubtedly subjective, however examples from nature provide simple rules to follow where no record of the natural teeth exist.

Materials used for the production of artificial teeth exhibit a range of mechanical properties and as such should be chosen to suit the patient requirements and the desired working life of the denture. Denture base material should also be chosen to suit the required strength and aesthetics.

Chapter 2 | PRE-PROSTHETIC TREATMENT

What's wrong with the old denture?

Fulfilling the requirements of function and aesthetics is challenging enough, so why not make use of the clues that exist before commencing work? Take a look at the existing denture.

Assess the denture's retention

- Has it gradually deteriorated?
- Is the extension of the denture correct?
- Is there a continuous border seal?
- Is there any mobile mucosa?

Is it stable?

- Is the occlusal table optimally designed?
- Are the teeth in the neutral zone?
- Are there any premature contacts on closing?
- Is the patient functioning from centric relation?
- Is there a balanced occlusion?
- Is there stability in protrusion?

How does it work aesthetically?

- Should the anterior aesthetics be duplicated?
- Is there significant wear?
- Has the patient ever liked it?
- Is there a record of the natural teeth?
- Is the vertical dimension correct?

Techniques in Complete Denture Technology, First Edition. Tony Johnson, Duncan J. Wood.
© 2012 Tony Johnson and Duncan J. Wood. Published 2012 by Blackwell Publishing Ltd.

How well does it function?

- Is the patient comfortable, stable and functioning from centric relation?
- Is the vertical dimension correct and will any increase be tolerated?

When assessing an existing denture, some features will be simple and quick to assess, confirm or even correct. Others may require further investigation prior to undertaking the task of producing a denture.

Modifying the denture

Modifying an existing denture to correct basic errors, test new positions or dimensions may be possible even if a number of problems exist. Alternatively, a copy of the existing denture can be made and the modifications tried out on this.

The following simple adjustments can be tried to diagnose problems with retention, stability, function and aesthetics.

Retention

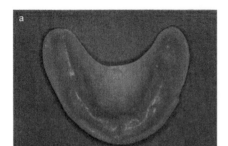

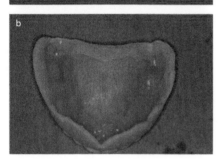

Figure 1

- Extend the denture base to cover the entire denture-bearing area chairside using light-curing material such as Triad VLC. Figure 1a shows an inadequately extended denture and Figure 1b shows extension provided with autopolymerising polymethyl methacrylate (PMMA) resin.
- If the the extension is satisfactory it can be relined either chairside or via the laboratory.

Stability

- Remove premature contacts and establish balanced occlusion. Premature contacts are easily removed chairside; establishing a balanced occlusion may require a check-record procedure on an articulator.
- Decrease the occlusal table by removing the most posterior teeth. This will help in several ways. First, there are fewer tooth contacts to establish, making the dentures easier to adjust. Second, there is less risk of the masticatory contacts being over the slope of the alveolar, which may be acting to dislodge the denture. As shown in Figure 2, leaving off the last molars that would be placed over the sloping parts of the lower ridges will improve stability. Finally, the contacts are further away from the condyles, which allows a greater tolerance when adjusting contacts (i.e. less accuracy is required).

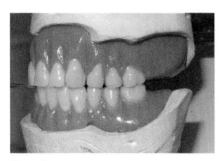

Figure 2

Function

- Increase the vertical dimension on existing dentures. This may serve two purposes. First, it may allow muscles to relax and the condyles to seat optimally in centric relation. If a patient has been posturing forwards, the lateral pterygoid muscle may shorten and allow the disc to fill the space behind the condylar head. Second, if a large increase in vertical dimension is required, the 'new' dimension may be tested prior to commencing treatment.

- Use self-curing acrylic on the occlusal surfaces of the teeth (premolar and molar only) to create an open bite. This could also be corrected using copy dentures. In Figure 3a, worn posterior teeth have created an over closed appearance. A trial temporary vertical dimension can be provided using autopolymerising PMMA resin placed onto the premolar and molar teeth as shown in Figure 3b,c.

Aesthetics

- Use modelling wax. It is difficult to show a patient what can be achieved with a denture without actually making a trail denture. The effect of increase in vertical dimension and additional lip support or tooth length can be demonstrated with the addition of modelling wax to the existing denture, but the results are limited.

- Have mould guides available. Having mould guides available in conjunction with a good-quality working mould guide as shown in Figure 4 may help. A three-dimensional mould guide provides the clinician and patient with the best opportunity to select the correct teeth required and seeing the various mould options arranged in different ways can be very helpful for both patients and clinicians when deciding upon the aesthetics required. Remember that pictures of the teeth options shown in mould guides (Figures 4b,c) are useful but never as good as looking at a set of the actual teeth in a working mould guide (Figure 4a). The best demonstration is to have some case studies available for the patient to see.

- Identify any presenting problems at an early stage, discussing the limitations will help set realistic expectations for the final dentures.

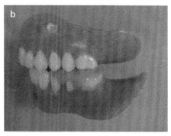
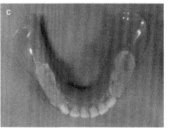
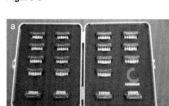

Figure 3

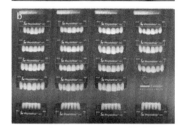
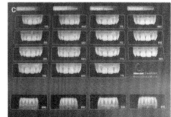

Figure 4

Chapter 3 | ACHIEVING A GOOD WORKING MODEL

Can I work with primary models?

Primary impressions in stock trays always cause overextension of the denture-bearing area because the impression material is displaced into the sulci. Figure 5 compares an overextended primary model (right) and a correctly extended (left) working model of the same mouth from an impression taken in a custom-made tray. Accurate recording of the functional sulcus is essential to define the denture extension and resulting retention and stability. Retention depends on the denture extending to fill the sulcus and thus creating a seal; if the denture is overextended, stability is compromised and the muscles may be displaced.

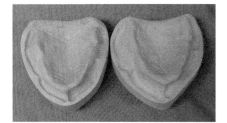

Figure 5

The excessive thickness of the material used in primary impressions results in poor accuracy both because of the amount of contraction on setting and over time and because of distortion resulting from the differing thickness of the material over the impression.

To achieve a good-quality working impression, it is essential to use a well-designed customised tray in conjunction with the appropriate impression material. This chapter explores the factors that govern choices in the design of tray and impression materials used.

Designing a customised impression tray

A customised impression tray should:

- allow easy control of the impression material;

- guide the impression material to the mucosa;

- support the impression material to provide even contact with the oral tissues;

- enable pressure on selected areas of the denture-bearing area;

- provide an even layer of impression material;

- support the set impression material;

- be rigid and retain its shape throughout the impression procedure and during the pouring of the model.

Techniques in Complete Denture Technology, First Edition. Tony Johnson, Duncan J. Wood.
© 2012 Tony Johnson and Duncan J. Wood. Published 2012 by Blackwell Publishing Ltd.

The design of the tray should ensure that:

- the tray is rigid;
- the entire denture-bearing area is included;
- the periphery of the tray finishes such that impression material can flow into the buccal and labial sulci without causing displacement of the soft tissues;
- the tray is spaced appropriately for the amount of undercut present;
- the handle is designed to avoid displacing the lips;
- the tray allows free movement of any muscle attachments.

Selecting an impression tray and material

In selecting an impression tray and material, the primary considerations are the amount of undercut present and whether any areas of the mucosa are mobile or unsupported.

Close-fitting trays

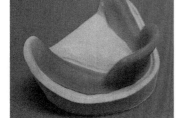
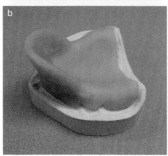

Where the majority of the denture-bearing area is free from large undercuts, close-fitting trays should be used (Figure 6a,b). These are ideal because they allow pressure to be exerted on the denture-bearing area during the impression-taking procedure. Compressing the mucosa and 'adapting' the relaxed mucosal tissue closely to the underlying alveolar bone helps in that the resultant fitting surface of the denture mirrors that of the mucosa under load during function. This allows the masticatory forces acting on the denture to be transmitted directly and comfortably to the alveolar bone.

The impression materials used with these trays are mucostatic in nature, however when used in thin section with close-fitting trays, the impression technique produces mucocompressive impressions. In addition, close-fitting trays allow a thin, uniform layer of impression material to be used. Thin sections of material are beneficial as shrinkage on setting or over time is minimal.

As there are only small amounts of undercut present, close-fitting impression trays such as those seen in Figure 6 may be used with impression materials that are non-elastic or rigid once set, typically zinc oxide and eugenol paste. Where these are unavailable, a medium-bodied silicone material may be used.

Figure 6

Spaced trays

Large undercut areas prohibit the use of close-fitting trays as removal from the mouth without causing distortion would be difficult and removal from the cast model would cause fracture of the cast. The spacing between the tray and the tissues should be increased according to the depth of undercut, tear strength and elastic limit of the impression material. In short, the greater the depth of the undercut, the more likely the material is to tear or exceed its elastic limit on removal.

Table 1 Space requirement for impression materials

Impression material	Space required
Zinc oxide and eugenol paste	No spacer wax (0.5–1 mm)
Silicone (medium bodied)	1.5–3 mm (one layer of wax)
Alginate	3 mm (two layers of wax)
Silicone (heavy bodied)	3–4.5 mm (three layers of wax)
Impression plaster	4.5 mm (three layers of wax)

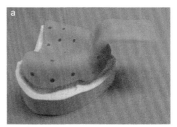
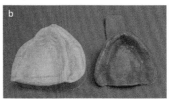
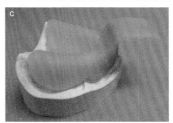

The solution is to provide greater spacing where large undercuts are present. Similarly a weak material such as alginate requires greater thickness than a tough material like silicone. Figure 7a shows a perforated spaced tray for use with alginate impression material and Figure 7b the wax spacer used to provide room for the impression material between the impression tray and the mouth. The amount of spacer required depends on the tear strength of the impression material being used: the weaker the material the thicker the spacer required. Figure 7c shows a spaced tray for use with silicone type impression material. No perforations are needed for this type of impression material.

One further consideration is the viscosity of the unset impression material (Table 1); if it is very high, additional spacing is necessary to allow seating of the tray without using excessive force. The use of such high-viscosity materials is rarely indicated in complete denture prosthetics.

Figure 7

Windowed trays

Where fibrous ridges are present, impression techniques must be adapted to ensure that the mobile tissue is not displaced during the recording procedure. In this circumstance, the impression is taken in two stages using a customised tray designed such that there is a 'window' over the fibrous ridge as shown in Figure 8.

First, a close-fitting impression is taken over the denture-bearing area in a modified tray using a zinc oxide/eugenol impression material. Once set, a second mucostatic material can be used to record the mobile area. Impression plaster is ideal as it can be applied without causing distortion and readily adheres to the impression tray. Alternatively, low-viscosity silicone may be used.

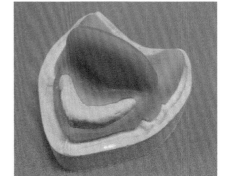

Figure 8

Producing customised trays

Identifying the peripheral extension

The extent of the customised tray should be determined with the patient present and recorded on to the primary impression. The simplest method is to mark the extension with an indelible pencil on the alginate impression, which subsequently 'tattoos' onto the primary model (Figure 9); use a permanent marker pen on silicone materials. If convenient, the required peripheral outline may be drawn directly onto the model.

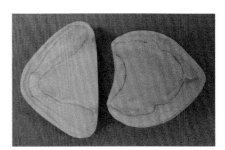

Figure 9

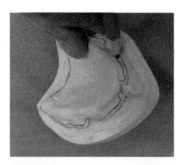

Figure 10

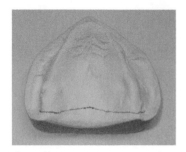

Figure 11

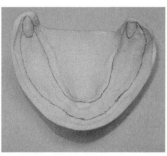

Figure 12

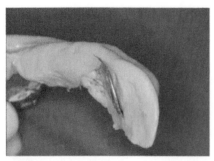

Figure 13

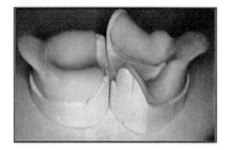

Figure 14

An approximation of the peripheral extension may be made using the primary model. The simplest method is to identify the deepest part of the sulcus, then draw the proposed periphery relative to this, taking into account the thickness of the impression material. This allows room for the material to wrap around the periphery of the tray.

For a 1.5-mm spaced tray, draw the extent of the tray 1.5 mm toward the alveolar ridge from the deepest part of the sulcus as shown in Figure 10. The tray periphery should be made slightly short of the required denture extension to allow room for the impression material being used. Draw the extension to avoid any muscle attachments here and double the space for the impression material on each side of the attachment.

For the maxillae, identify the junction between the hard and soft palate (foveae palatine) and use this landmark as the periphery of the tray, ensuring that the entire tuberosities are included. As shown in Figure 11, the distal extension of maxillary impression trays should extend to the foveae palatine and extend beyond the tuberosities to the hamular notches.

For the mandible, include the retromolar pad and extend into the lingual sulcus such that the periphery is just short of the mylohyoid ridge and buccally to be just short of the external oblique ridge, as shown in Figure 12.

Prescription information

Any prescription should include the following information.

- The type of impression material that will be used for the working impression.
- The type of tray required.
- The amount of spacer wax required.
- An indication of the peripheral extension of the tray, taking into account the thickness of the impression material to be used.
- Any special features required (outline window tray positions and whether a variable thickness of spacer wax is required).
- Type of handle required (intraoral, extraoral, finger stops, stepped or not and where the handle for a windowed tray should be placed).

Design of a close-fitting tray

This type of tray is used with zinc oxide/eugenol impression paste low-viscosity impression materials. The close fit allows the fluid impression materials to be controlled in a thin layer and to locate precisely against the ridge.

Care should be taken to ensure that the tray extends to the required depth of the sulcus; where short, the mechanically weak impression materials will be unsupported and susceptible to distortion. Figure 13, for example, shows an inadequately supported impression. It has become detached from the tray and would be likely to distort during model preparation.

If overextended, the tray will displace the muscle insertions and lead to an inaccurate impression. The customised impression trays shown in Figure 14 are obviously overextended and will lead to inaccurate impressions if not extensively adjusted by the clinician.

Close-fitting trays should be thin at the periphery to prevent the sulcus becoming overloaded with impression material and to allow room for the impression material to fully mould around this area of the tray without the tray 'pushing' the material away during impression taking (Figure 15a,b).

Excess impression material or a thick tray will cause displacement of the soft tissues, resulting in a false record of the sulcus. It is worth bearing in mind that the alveolar suffers little resorption in these areas. In the overextended impressions shown in Figure 16, the sulcus and muscle attachment sites are distorted.

The handles for close-fitting trays are best designed to be intraoral as shown in Figure 17. In this position, the labial aspect of the handle supports the lip in a natural manner, avoiding distortion of the labial sulcus. The height of the handle should be such that it is level with the top of the lip and it should extend distally around the ridge to the premolar region. This allows the clinician's fingers to exert pressure on the baseplate evenly along the entire impression tray after seating the impression, as shown in Figure 18.

Design of a close-fitting windowed tray

There are occasions when a close-fitting custom tray would be desirable, but is contraindicated by the presence of a fibrous ridge, as shown in Figure 19. These fibrous ridges need not always preclude the use of a close-fitting custom tray zinc oxide/eugenol paste impression being taken. The problem can be overcome by the use of a close-fitting tray with a window cut in the tray around the fibrous ridge area (Figure 20), allowing the firm parts of the ridge to be recorded in zinc oxide/eugenol paste and the fibrous part to be recorded in a more fluid material.

In these cases, tray handles are placed across the centre of the palate for maxillary cases, allowing the anterior region to be left open. For mandibular trays, finger stops are placed where they will not interfere with the window, as shown in Figure 21.

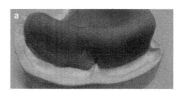
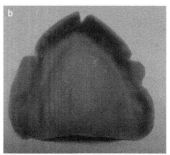

Figure 15

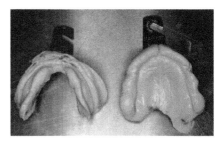

Figure 16

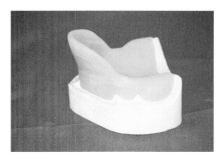

Figure 17

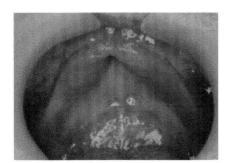

Figure 19

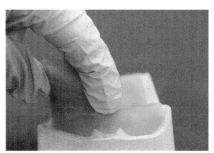

Figure 18

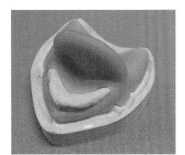

Figure 20

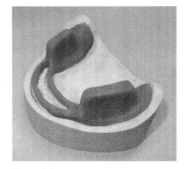

Figure 21

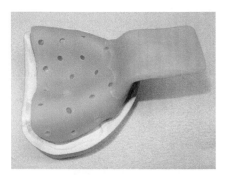

Figure 22

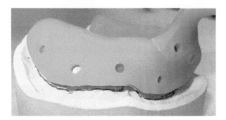

Figure 23

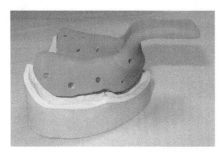

Figure 24

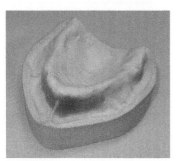

Figure 25

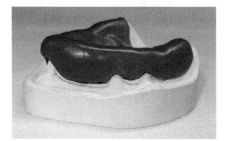

Figure 26

Design of a spaced tray

This type of custom tray can be used with alginate, elastomeric and impression plaster impression materials.

Alginate has low tear strength and requires adequate bulk to remain intact on removal. In addition, when recording large undercuts the impression material must be thick enough to prevent distortion on removal of the set material by exceeding its elastic limit. Trays for alginate are perforated to allow mechanical retention to retain alginate in the tray, as shown in Figure 22.

The tray spacing extends to 1–2 mm short of the periphery, with the exception of the post-dam region. This allows the impression material to flow around the tray periphery and record the sulcus. As shown in Figure 23, it is important not to place the perforations too close to the edge of the tray. If the clinician needs to adjust any overextension of the tray they may grind into the perforations.

An extraoral handle is placed anteriorly and includes a step to ensure that it exits the mouth between the lips without displacing them (Figure 24).

Model preparation

For close-fitting custom trays, any undercuts should be filled with modelling wax, as shown in Figure 25. This ensures that the tray can be removed from the model and from the working model after casting.

If the tray is to be spaced, adapt the appropriate thickness of modelling wax to the model and trim short of the required peripheral depth required for the impression material to be used prior to tray construction (see Table 1; Figure 26).

Tray base construction

1. Coat the exposed plaster surfaces with separating solution to prevent the tray material sticking to the model.

2. Adapt the light-curing blank to the model, or over the wax spacer, taking care to avoid thinning the material, as shown in Figure 27. The blanks are provided at the required thickness to ensure the tray is rigid during use.

3. Trim the excess material with a wax knife to the required peripheral extension. The final extension can be ground using a tungsten carbide bur and micromotor (Figures 28a,b).

Handle construction

Intraoral: for use with close-fitting custom trays

1. Form a rectangular shape approximately 2 × 6 cm and 3–4 mm thick. Adapt this to fit over the crest of the anterior ridge, extending to the premolar region. The anterior section of the handle should replicate the contour of the missing anterior teeth and, as shown in Figure 29, should be shaped to support the lips in as natural a position as possible to aid accurate impression taking around the labial sulcus.

2. Press the handle material firmly against the base to blend the material. Vaseline is useful to smooth the join between hard and soft material (Figure 30).

3. Trim to create a curved handle that guides the fingers to the centre of the tray, allowing even pressure to be exerted over the entire tray base during impression taking (Figure 31a,b).

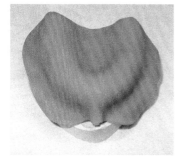

Figure 27

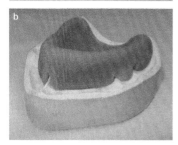

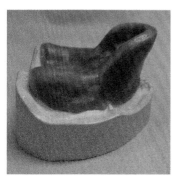

Figure 28

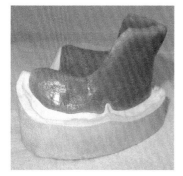

Figure 29

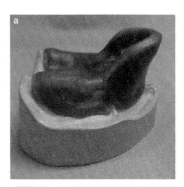

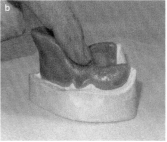

Figure 31

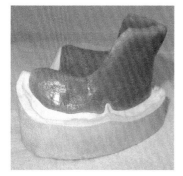

Figure 30

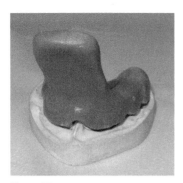

Figure 32

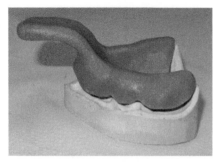

Figure 33

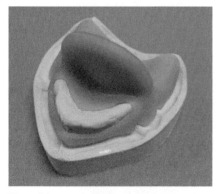

Figure 34

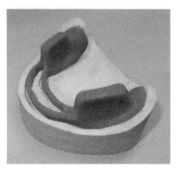

Figure 35

Extraoral: for use with spaced custom trays

1. Form a rectangle approximately 5 × 2.5 cm and 3–4 mm thick. Adapt one end to the anterior ridge across the mid-line and blend into the base as previously described (Figure 32).

2. Make a right-angled bend approximately 1.5 cm from the tray base to form a step in the handle (Figure 33) to ensure that the handle exits between the lips and does not distort the commissure of the lips during impression taking.

Intraoral: for use with windowed trays

For maxillary trays, attach a rectangle of material 3 × 4 cm and 3–4 mm thick across the palate in the premolar region, as shown in Figure 34.

For mandibular trays, place finger stops away from any fibrous ridge sites (Figure 35). To achieve a more secure bond between the base and handle these two parts of the tray can be made together before light curing, as described above.

Finishing the tray

Ensure that the tray is strong and rigid enough by adding material where appropriate. This is particularly important for large lower trays, where silicone is to be used. Figure 36a shows a mandibular tray with long posterior sections that could be rather weak. These can be strengthened by placing extra material along their length as shown in Figure 36b.

If the tray is to be used with alginate, 2-mm holes should be drilled in the base material after curing. The holes should be 10 mm apart and finish 3–4 mm from the periphery of the tray (Figure 37). This allows chairside adjustment of the periphery without risk of grinding into the holes.

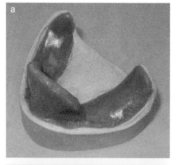

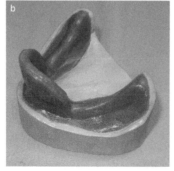

Figure 36

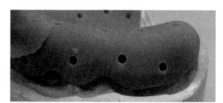

Figure 37

Once smooth, the material is cured by placing in an ultraviolet (UV) light box. The curing process usually takes approximately 2 minutes; however the light source may not cure the full depth of the material, particularly underneath the handle. Therefore it should be removed carefully and the curing cycle repeated with the tray inverted and any wax removed.

Trim to shape with tungsten carbide burs. Final smoothing may be achieved using a sandpaper mandrel and sandpaper strips. Extra grip on the handle can be provided by grinding retention grooves across the handle, as shown in Figure 38, using a small tungsten carbide bur.

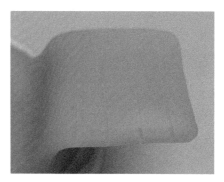

Figure 38

Custom trays that have been smoothed with sandpaper can sometimes look a little rough (Figure 39 left). The appearance of the tray can be improved by rubbing Vaseline into the surface of the tray and then light-curing in the UV light box (Figure 39 centre). Hot water or a solvent should then be used to remove any excess Vaseline. Alternatively, commercially produced light-curing varnishes can also be purchased and applied (Figure 39 right).

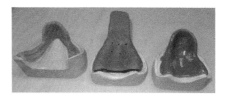

Figure 39

Secondary impressions and working models

Close fitting

When using close-fitting trays, the extension should be checked and adjusted chairside. First check the tray on the primary model. Particular attention should be paid to the frenal attachments to and distal extension of the tray.

To check in the patient's mouth, lightly hold the tray in position and manipulate the lips and cheeks in an attempt to displace the tray. For the lower tray, ask the patient to lift the tongue to check the lingual extension.

Where a tray is short, light-curing composite material or impression compound may be added. This should then be border moulded in the mouth while soft.

When using zinc oxide/eugenol paste (ZOE), a thin, even layer should be applied across the entire tray and around the periphery. When taking the impression, apply an even, gentle force to allow the material to slowly flow into position. Check that the material flows into the sulci and out of the distal of the tray. Manipulate the lips and cheeks as before to create a function recording of the attachments and sulic. Ask the patient to push the tongue forward when taking the lower impression to shape the impression material in the lingual sulcus.

Using a low-viscosity silicone impression material in a close fitting tray requires a tray adhesive to be carefully applied. Be aware that the materials will be in very thin section and, if not adhered adequately to the tray, is susceptible to tearing.

Casting a model from a zinc oxide/eugenol close-fitting impression

When casting models from this type of impression, care should be taken to ensure that the tray periphery does not get encased in plaster. Marking a line around the periphery using a permanent marker pen as shown in Figure 40 can be very useful when casting.

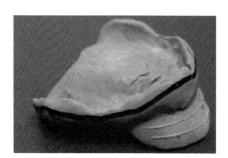

Figure 40

To remove the impression from the cast, soften the zinc oxide/eugenol paste by immersing in warm water for 2–3 minutes. The material should leave the model cleanly. Overheating the material will result in residual material adhering to the cast.

Spaced trays

The extension of the tray must be checked as for close-fitting trays, with the knowledge that adequate room is required for the extra thickness of material. Again, particular attention should be given to the muscle insertion areas.

If the tray has perforations for alginate material, ensure that the tray is not weakened on adjustment of the periphery.

Windowed trays

The first stage of taking the impression with zinc oxide/eugenol paste is the same as described for close-fitting trays.

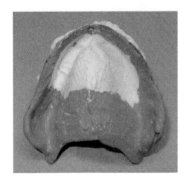

Figure 41

1. Once you are happy with the impression of the firm parts of the ridges, trim the zinc oxide/eugenol paste back to the window edge.

2. Re-insert the impression and apply the same constant pressure as when taking the zinc oxide/eugenol paste impression.

3. Apply the impression plaster over the mobile area using a brush, gradually increasing the thickness. Once set, remove the impression (Figure 41).

4. To cast this model, apply a separator to the impression plaster before casting.

5. Once the model is fully set, remove the plaster by making gentle taps with a small hammer.

6. Warm the zinc oxide/eugenol paste as previously described to remove the remainder of the impression.

7. Low-viscosity silicone may be used as an alternative to impression plaster.

Chapter 4 | OCCLUSAL REGISTRATION

Introduction

The occlusal registration stage records the information required to produce the trial dentures. There are five essential recordings made: occlusal plane, centre line, lip support, vertical dimension and centric relation.

Further information indicating tooth position may also be recorded, such as smile lines and canine lines or helpful techniques such as neutral zone recording.

Anatomical relationships may be recorded to correctly position models on the articulator using a facebow registration, and gothic arch tracing may be used to ascertain centric relation.

This chapter will discuss the design and use of occlusal registration rims to record this information.

Design of registration rims

Although the baseplate and wax rim together replace the teeth and any resorbed alveolar bone, registration rims are often constructed without specific aim or method and with little consideration for anatomical features.

Production of rims on primary models is not advocated. It is rare for rims produced on a primary model to fit working casts accurately. The anatomical features recorded on the secondary impression, such as the sulcus width and depth, should be used to design the registration rim.

A well-designed registration rim is quick and easy to construct and saves time during both the clinical registration stage and the production of the trial dentures.

It should be remembered, however, that a problem with all rims is that they will not demonstrate the potential retention expected from the finished dentures. This is because they are produced on blocked-out working models as shown in Figure 42. If the baseplates were made on the working models without blocking out undercuts, the model would be damaged during the frequent removal of the rims from the models during denture construction.

In constructing registration rims there are three design considerations:

* baseplate rigidity and extension;

* anterior and posterior rim width; and

* anterior and posterior rim height.

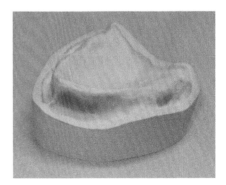

Figure 42

Techniques in Complete Denture Technology, First Edition. Tony Johnson, Duncan J. Wood.
© 2012 Tony Johnson and Duncan J. Wood. Published 2012 by Blackwell Publishing Ltd.

Baseplate rigidity and extension

A baseplate should be rigid, dimensionally stable at working temperatures and extend over the entire denture-bearing area. Baseplates are commonly constructed from wax, shellac or light-cured acrylic. To be dimensionally stable, rigid enough at the desired thickness, and to allow adjustment to the periphery chairside, light-cured acrylic is the most suitable material. If wax or shellac are used, consideration should be given to the possible distortion in the mouth due to an increase in temperature.

The techniques for denture production described in the following chapters will use rigid light-cured acrylic baseplate for the construction of the registration rims for the trial dentures. The rigid baseplate also allows the registration rim to be used without modification for gothic arch tracing and facebow registration. The time taken to produce a well-designed baseplate from light-cured acrylic is a sound investment and takes no longer than producing a baseplate from shellac.

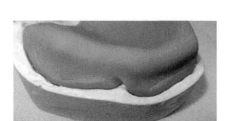

Figure 43

The buccal and labial sulcus and the junction of the hard and soft palate determine the extension of the maxillary baseplate. The peripheral border of the baseplate should fill the sulcus and be shaped to allow free movement of any muscle attachments. If the working impression has been correctly extended and the periphery border moulded, the registration rim base should completely fill the sulcus area of the model as shown in Figure 43.

If possible, it is beneficial to cut a post dam at this stage to provide improved retention of the registration rim. Post dams are cut using a chisel such that they are deeper towards the soft palate. They should extend beyond the hamular notches and into the buccal sulcus and be broader and get deeper towards the soft palate as shown in Figure 44. The clinician, who should have assessed the depth of tissue in this area, should ideally cut them.

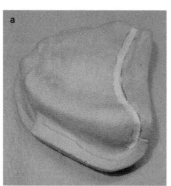

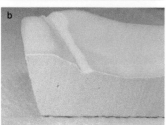

Figure 44

The post dam should enclose the tuberosities and end in the buccal sulcus. The depth of the dam, typically 1–2 mm, is determined by the mucosa, and where only thin layers of mucosa are present across the midline, the depth is reduced to 1 mm.

The baseplate material is approximately 1.5 mm thick and therefore should require little shaping, however consideration of the bone loss adjacent to the periphery is required, particularly in the labial region where little bone loss occurs. The baseplate should be thinned to prevent any displacement of soft tissue.

The mandibular baseplate follows similar criteria, however it should finish at the distal edge of the retromolar pad, and lingually should be shaped to provide as much room for the tongue as possible.

Anterior and posterior rim width

Rim width is an important feature that can contribute to the ease of the clinical registration stage. Adjustment of the rims is quicker and easier with narrower rims.

Rims should be slightly wider than the teeth they will eventually carry (i.e. approximately 8–9 mm in the molar region and 5–6 mm across the midline (Figure 45).

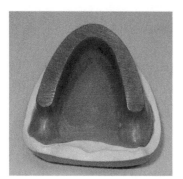

Figure 45

Wide rims restrict tongue space and displace the cheeks and lips. This is likely to result in difficulties in assessing lip support, aesthetics and phonetics or vertical dimension. Displacing soft tissues may also break the peripheral seal, resulting in poor retention and/or movement of the registration rims.

Anterior and posterior rim height

The height of the rim should be made to average dimensions and the occlusal plane angled to conform to the ala-tragal (or Camper's) line to ensure minimal adjustment is necessary during the registration stage.

The average height of the maxillary rim, measured from the lowest point of the labial sulcus next to the central frenum to the top of the registration rim, should be 22 mm (Figure 46). This dimension is indicated by studies that have measured both natural teeth and adjusted rims after the occlusal registration stage. Paying attention to this detail in the laboratory results in the minimal amount of adjustment being required chairside.

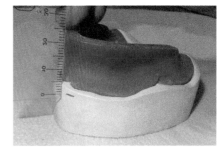

Figure 46

An alternative method is to copy the vertical dimension from existing dentures using an Alma gauge as shown in Figure 47. This device uses the incisal papillae as a reference point and allows vertical height to be measured and reproduced, as well as the labial contour.

Once occlusal rim height is established, the occlusal plane is determined using an occlusal plane inclinator. As shown in Figure 48, this instrument has a lip on the posterior border which is placed across the hamular notches and 'folded' down towards the reference height while maintaining contact with the baseplate. To use it, the rim inclinator is heated, the back edge placed across the hamular notches and the hot plate brought into contact with the wax rim until the wax has melted away to the 22 mm mark at the front (Figure 49).

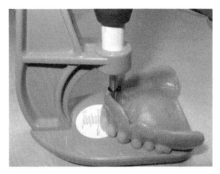

Figure 47

This procedure provides an approximation of the occlusal plane as it rises from the incisors to the molars along the curve of Spee, parallel to the ala-tragal (or Camper's) line (Figure 50).

The average height of the mandibular rim, measured from the lowest point of the sulcus next to the central frenum, should be 18 mm (Figure 51), and the occlusal plane should be adjusted such that the posterior height is two-thirds the way up the retromolar pad at the back (Figure 52). The rim should extend posteriorly to the region of the second molar teeth.

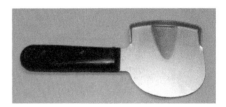

Figure 48

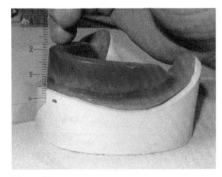

Figure 51

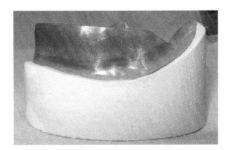

Figure 52

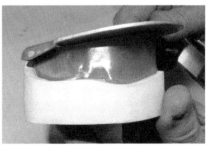

Figure 49

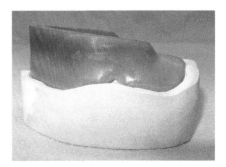

Figure 50

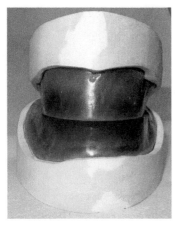

Figure 53

The contour of the wax between the peripheral border and the occlusal plane should replace any lost alveolar and harness the retentive forces of the soft tissues. This is achieved by building the buccal aspect such that it contacts the cheek without displacing it, creating a better peripheral seal and allowing the muscles to act with the polished surface to seat the rim (Figure 53).

Construction of registration rims

1. Fill any undercut areas on the model with molten modelling wax and coat the exposed plaster with plaster separating solution (Figure 54).

2. Adapt a light-curing blank closely to the model, trimming away the excess to reveal the land area of the model. The base should extend to fill the entire sulcus. Roughen the crests of the bases to aid retention of the wax rims. Smooth using Vaseline and cure. Remember that it can be difficult to obtain a retentive bond between the light-curing acrylic resin base material and the wax rims. Mechanical retentive grooves placed into the bases before curing, as shown in Figure 55, can improve the bond significantly.

3. Trim with a tungsten carbide bur and use sandpaper to smooth the periphery. Vaseline can be used to improve the appearance of the base if necessary.

4. A small amount of molten sticky wax may be placed onto the crests of the bases to further aid in the retention of the wax rims. Pass the flame of a Bunsen burner over the sticky wax to melt it prior to placing the wax rim.

5. Soften a wax rim in warm water (40–45°C) until pliable, dry it, and then slightly melt the underside with a Bunsen flame and immediately place onto the base. Adapt the wax rim tightly onto the base using the fingers and thumb (Figure 56a,b).

6. Ensure the labial surface is correctly aligned 10 mm forward of the incisal papillae on the maxillary base and over the centre of the ridge on the mandibular base.

7. Using a hot wax knife seal the edges of the wax rim to the base with modelling wax (Figure 57).

8. Draw a pencil mark on the outside of the model to be level with the lowest point of the sulcus next to the central frenum (Figure 58).

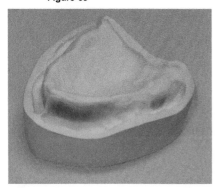

Figure 54

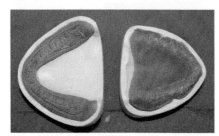

Figure 55

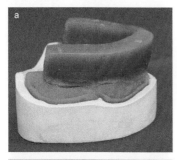
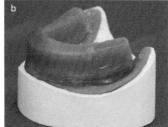

Figure 56

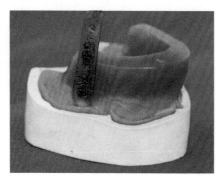

Figure 57

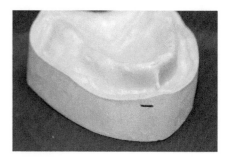

Figure 58

9. Measure from this mark 18–19 mm for the mandibular rim and 22–23 mm for the maxillary rim and mark the wax rims with a wax knife at these points (Figure 59a,b). It is a good idea to add 1 mm to these measurements to allow for finishing the surface of the rim later in the process.

10. Use an occlusal rim inclinator placed across the hamular notches to form the antero-posterior angle of the maxillary block. Heat the plate over a Bunsen burner then place the back edge of the plate onto the hamular notches. Bring the hot plate down against the wax rim and start to melt away the excess wax (Figure 60).

11. Remember that the hamular notches are never level so select the highest to contact to ensure that you do not build a slope into the rim surface.

12. When the desired height at the front of the rim is reached (22–23 mm), you will have created the average antero-posterior slope on the surface of the rim (Figure 61).

13. Adjust the mandibular rim in height to be 18–19 mm anteriorly and for the rims to be level with a point two-thirds the way up the retromolar pads as marked in Figure 62a,b.

14. A line can be drawn in the wax between these two points with a wax knife and the excess wax removed using a hot wax knife or using the occlusal rim inclinator as a hot plate.

15. Adjust the rim width to be approximately 5–6 mm anteriorly and 8–9 mm posteriorly.

16. Finish the wax surface with a flame or wax solvent to a smooth surface.

17. Finally, score the rims across a piece of sandpaper on a flat surface to level the tops and polish the surface of the wax with liquid soap and cotton wool to leave the rims meeting evenly and highly polished (Figure 63).

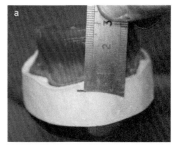
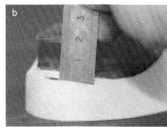

Figure 59

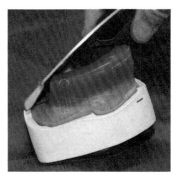

Figure 60

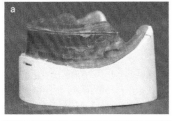
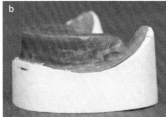

Figure 62

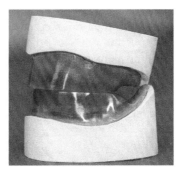

Figure 63

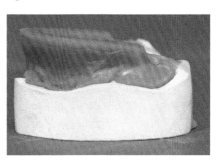

Figure 61

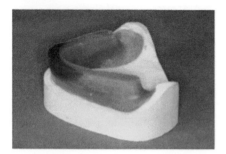

Figure 64

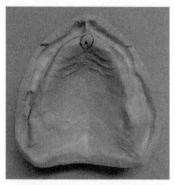

Figure 65

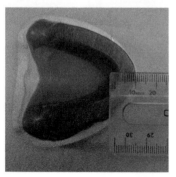

Figure 66

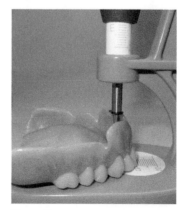

Figure 67

Occlusal registration

Occlusal plane and lip support

The occlusal plane is the plane at which the upper and lower teeth occlude. It passes through the incisal edge of the central incisors and curves upwards as it travels towards the molars (curve of Spee). Figure 64 shows the teeth set to conform to the curve of Spee.

The occlusal plane is significant in providing suitable aesthetics, phonetics and function for the dentures. The incisal edge of the central incisors is the primary determinant for establishing the occlusal plane in edentulous cases. The labial surfaces of the anterior teeth or rim also provide support for the lips. Figure 65 shows how wax added to the labial surface of a mandibular block to support the lips can be used to achieve the correct labial contour to the face. Either adding or removing wax from the labial surface of the rim until the angle between the columella of the nose, and the upper lip approximates a right angle can achieve this.

The desired position is determined using a combination of anatomical landmarks, aesthetics and phonetics. Positioning of the anterior teeth at this stage allows the aesthetics and phonetics to be assessed more readily. To do this the correct mould shape and size of tooth should be chosen.

Anatomical landmarks

The incisal papillae may be used to assess the position of the labial surface of central incisors, which are typically 9–10 mm anterior to the middle of the incisal papillae. This can be measured on a model by drawing a line through the papillae at right angles to the midline and marking this on the land area or the model as shown in Figure 66.

The registration rim can then be positioned and the line drawn onto the occlusal plane of the rim. Now the labial surface can be shaped such that it falls 10 mm anteriorly, providing lip support, as shown in Figure 67.

There is a specifically designed measuring tool, which allows this to be carried out more quickly. The Alma gauge (Figure 68) uses the incisal papillae as a reference position and allows the labial contour to be measured, recorded and copied. The device also allows the vertical dimension to be assessed in relation to the incisal papillae.

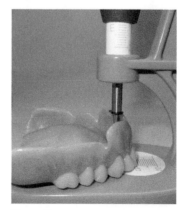

Figure 68

Aesthetics

Looking at the soft tissues around the top lip can help to assess the labial positioning. The patient should have a natural profile. With the lip at rest, the amount of tooth or rim visible is used to determine the vertical height of the occlusal plane. The amount of tooth or rim showing will differ for each patient, just as it does when teeth are present. The best aid is a photograph of the patient when dentate, or with a denture that they liked.

When attempting to establish the most favourable position, consider the skeletal classification, the age of the patient and existing denture. It should be remembered that an elderly person would naturally show fewer teeth below a relaxed upper lip than a young person.

The skeletal relationships of the mandible to the maxilla will inevitably alter the relationship between the mandibular and maxillary teeth.

Figures 69 shows the expected relationship between the posterior teeth for a class I relationship. Figure 70 shows the same for the anterior teeth, including a typical 2 mm overbite and overjet. As shown in Figure 71, in class II denture cases the maxillary posterior teeth usually exhibit a greater buccal cusp overjet than that seen in class I cases. This is due to a skeletal relationship, where the mandible is positioned distally in relation to the maxilla. As shown in Figure 72, the maxillary anterior teeth in a class II skeletal relationship also exhibit a much larger overjet than is seen in class I cases.

In class III denture cases the situation is the reverse of that seen in the class II cases. This sees the mandible positioned anteriorly in relation to the maxilla. This usually sees the mandibular posterior teeth positioned buccally in relation to the maxillary teeth and is usually accompanied by a lateral or bilateral 'crossbite' arrangement of the teeth, as shown in Figure 73. The anterior teeth in class III cases usually have an 'edge-to-edge' relationship as shown in Figure 74. Sometimes it is even difficult to achieve even an 'edge-to-edge' relationship and still be able to keep the teeth over the ridges.

It should be noted that although the relationship of the posterior teeth to each other may alter laterally, depending on whether it is class II, buccal overjet, or class III, crossbite, the antero-posterior relationship of the maxillary and mandibular teeth remains the same for all three classifications.

Attempting to make skeletal class II and class III cases into class I cases often results in unstable dentures due to the teeth being positioned outside the ridges.

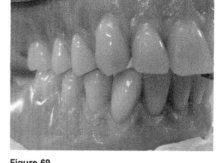

Figure 69

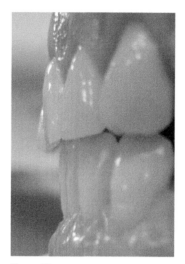

Figure 70

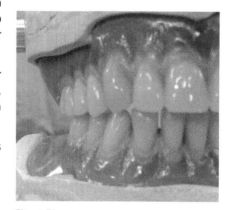

Figure 71

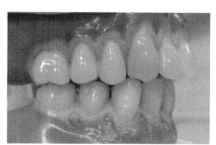

Figure 72

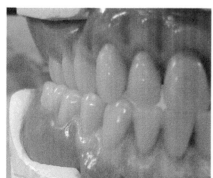

Figure 73

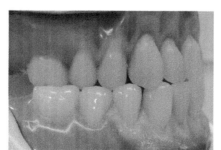

Figure 74

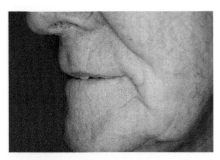

Figure 75

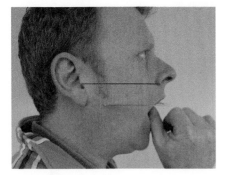

Figure 76

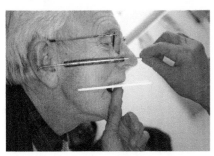

Figure 77

Phonetics

When 'F' is pronounced, the incisal edge of the maxillary incisors should just touch the wet–dry border of the lower lip (Figure 75). This can be used as a test of the position of the incisal edge.

Existing denture

An existing denture is an excellent guide when establishing the occlusal plane of the new denture. The position of the teeth can be measured using the Alma gauge and duplicated on the registration rim or new denture. Where necessary, this can be adjusted to improve the position.

Alternatively, a copy denture technique may be used (see *Basics of Dental Technology: a Step by Step Approach*, Chapter 2, page 62, ISBN 978-1-4051-7875-4, for a description of a copy denture technique).

Once the incisal determinant is established, the occlusal plane of the upper registration rim is adjusted to be parallel to the ala-tragal (or Camper's) line. This is a reference plane that is drawn between the inferior border of the ala of the nose and the superior border of the tragus of the ear and is approximately parallel to the occlusal plane of the natural teeth. Figure 76 shows one of the authors holding a Foxes occlusal plane indicator against his natural teeth. It can be seen that the occlusal plane of the natural teeth are parallel to the ala-tragal line.

A Foxes occlusal plane indicator held against the upper rim allows the occlusal plane to be viewed extraorally. At the same time, any handy straight implement can be held along the ala-tragal line to compare the reference plane to the occlusal plane of the upper rim, as shown in Figure 77.

Adjusting the upper rim

If the upper rim needs to be adjusted by removing wax from the rim, this can be achieved using a hot rim inclinator until the block is parallel with the reference plane.

If it is necessary to add wax to a rim, use the following procedure.

1. Cut off a piece of wax that will cover the rim.

2. Dry the occlusal rim.

3. Heat the wax in a flame, or hot air burner if working on the clinic, such that the surface melts a little.

4. Press this firmly onto the occlusal surface of the rim.

5. Using a very hot knife, cut around the rim through the wax sheet. If the knife cools it will drag the wax rather than cut it, therefore reheat regularly.

6. Heat the spoon end of the knife and use it to smooth the join by making a slow, even pass over the join.

7. Cool under running water.

Midline, smile line and canine line

The midline is marked on the upper rim in line with the midline of the face (Figure 78) unless harmony determines otherwise. When setting the anterior teeth chairside, any diastemma or desired tooth angle is set. Alternatively these details are noted on the prescription card to be carried out in the laboratory.

The smile and canine lines are useful in selecting the size of tooth to be placed. The height of the central incisor should be equal to or greater than the height of the smile line above the incisal edge (Figures 79a,b). Similarly, the distance between the canines can be determined from the corners of the mouth at rest. Marking these lines on the rim aids in the selection of tooth size.

Vertical dimensions

There are two vertical dimensions that are routinely measured: the occlusal face height when the teeth are in occlusion (Figure 80) and the rest face height when the mandible is in the rest position (Figure 81). For the production of dentures, the occlusal face height is recorded using the registration rims. The rest face height is used to help determine the occlusal face height.

To establish a functional vertical dimension the occlusal face height must be less than the rest face height to allow the occluding surfaces to separate at rest. The difference between the two is called the 'freeway space' and is significant because it allows the muscles of mastication periods of rest.

To establish an aesthetic vertical dimension, the occlusal face height should be such as to prevent large creases forming in the soft tissues at the corners of the mouth by being high enough, but must not be so high that the patient is incapable of forming an oral seal with the lips.

The rest face height is first determined using a Willis gauge (Figure 82a) or pair of dividers (Figure 82b). When using dividers, reference marks are positioned on the nose and chin.

The lower rim is adjusted such that it occludes evenly with the upper rim while allowing approximately 2–4 mm of freeway space (the minimum freeway space should be 2 mm, although in older patients it may be more than 4 mm).

The vertical dimension is now assessed for aesthetics and further reductions made as required. A useful starting point is to assess the patient with their existing dentures in place. If the occlusal height is satisfactory, it can be measured and established on the registration rims.

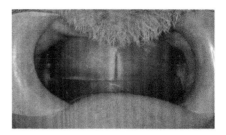

Figure 78

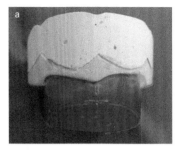

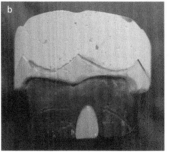

Figure 79

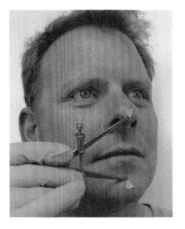

Figure 80

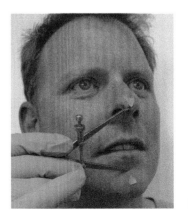

Figure 81

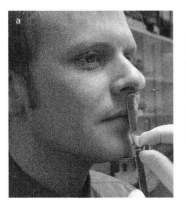

Figure 82

Lower lip support

The labial aspect of the lower rim is harmonised with the lower lip to ensure that the denture will remain seated during speech. A useful check is to ask the patient to pronounce the letter 'E', which pulls the lower lip against the labial aspect of the rim. Neutral zone techniques may be indicated in cases where positioning the lower rim or teeth is difficult (see Chapter 11, Special techniques, for a description of a neutral zone denture technique).

Centric relation

The centric relation is the relationship between the maxillae and mandible when the jaw is in its optimal position. For simplicity, this is when the condyle heads seat in the summit position of the glenoid fossa. In this position the mandible can hinge open approximately 15 mm without any forward movement of the condyles. Therefore centric relation can be described as a range of movement when the condyles are seated.

Centric relation is significant for several reasons.

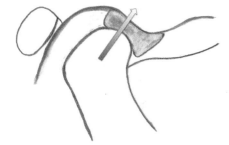

Figure 83

- It is the optimal position for load distribution: When force is transmitted through the mandible and into the temperomandibular joint, the forces are distributed through bony structures rather than being opposed by the musculature. This is therefore a comfortable position from which to function. Figure 83 shows the direction of the condyle head movement as forces are exerted in centric relation.

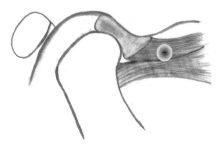

Figure 84

- It is the optimal position for muscle activity: Muscles act antagonistically and rely on periods of rest to avoid becoming fatigued. In centric relation the muscles can work antagonistically and prevent discomfort during function. Figure 84 shows the muscles working antagonistically in centric relation to prevent discomfort during function.

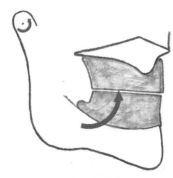

Figure 85

- It is the optimal position for repeatability: When producing a new inter-cuspal position for the patient a repeatable position is required to enable the occlusal contacts to be harmonised. With the mandible in centric relation, the jaw may be closed down to the correct vertical dimension on its hinge. This contact is termed retruded contact position (RCP). It is at this position that the new inter-cuspal position (ICP) will be established. Figure 85 shows the mandibular hinge action of the mandible down to the correct vertical dimension establishing the RCP.

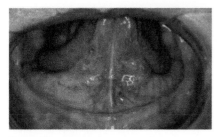

Figure 86

The most commonly used method to position the mandible in centric relation is to ask the patient to curl the tip of the tongue to the soft palate (Figure 86), encouraging the condyles to seat. While doing this, the mandible is closed to the RCP. If you try this yourself you will find that the position you close into is slightly more retruded than your normal ICP. See later in this section for a description of gothic arch tracing plates to see a method of recording a more relaxed RCP.

To check that the position is correct, the procedure is repeated several times and the positions compared to ensure they coincide. There is constant debate regarding the best, most reliable, accurate and repeatable techniques. A criticism of this one is that because it is not a 'natural' position it may lead to RCP being recorded 1–2 mm further posterior than expected when the activated muscles position the condyles.

To record this position, 'V'-shaped notches are cut into each rim and the exercise above repeated with silicone bite registration material between the rims (Figure 87).

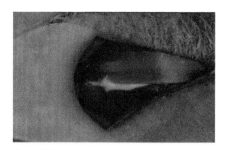

Figure 87

For patients deviating on closing, those with temporomandibular dysfunction (TMD) or simply if the normal procedure of recording RCP produces an uncomfortable position for the patient, the use of gothic arch tracing devices for locating and recording centric relation is indicated.

Gothic arch tracing

Gothic arch tracing (GAT) is a method of locating and recording centric relation using a horizontal tracing of the mandibular movements. To produce the tracing, a stylus is placed in the maxillary arch and a plate in the mandibular arch as shown in Figure 88. The patient is now asked to perform lateral and protrusive mandibular excursions, allowing the stylus to scribe its pathway on the plate. To allow this to be seen clearly, the plate is coloured with a wax crayon. A tracing like the one shown in Figure 89 is produced. The pattern resembles a gothic arch or arrowhead, giving rise to the name of the technique, although it may also be referred to as needlepoint tracing or central bearing point tracing.

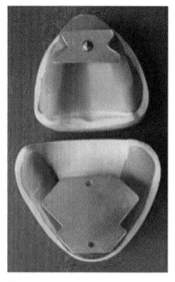

Figure 88

The tip of the arrow is formed where the excursions coincide (i.e. centric relation). It is this point that is used to make the final jaw registration. The mandible is 'held' in centric relation by the stylus entering a hole in a plastic disc located over the arrowhead as shown in Figure 90. The stylus should habitually locate into the hole in the plastic disc to confirm the correct relationship has been recorded (Figure 91).

Unlike the 'curl the tongue to the back of the palate' method, the GAT method records a completely relaxed position.

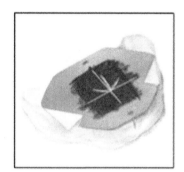

Figure 89

The registration of the jaw position is then made using silicone bite registration material or impression plaster between the registration rims (Figure 92).

This method of recording the relationship between the mandible and maxilla has the advantage that the centric relation position is verified at the jaw registration stage. These devices are usually intraoral and can be used to record centric relation in both dentate and edentulous patients. The technique may be used independently or in conjunction with a facebow; both of these approaches are described in the following text.

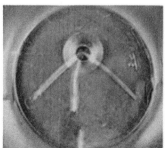

Figure 90

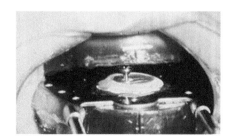

Figure 91

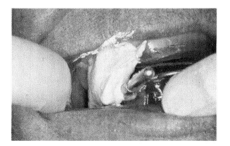

Figure 92

Gothic arch tracing device construction

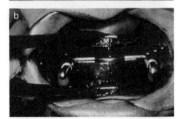

The tracing plate and stylus are placed onto the occlusal surfaces of the registration rims once the vertical dimension has been established and recorded. Well-constructed, correctly extended registration rims are essential for stability when carrying out this procedure. For precise recording, a piece of wire is inserted into the anterior labial surface of each rim (Figure 93a,b). The distance between the markers is measured with the rims together and this is then used to re-establish the correct vertical dimension once the stylus and plate have been positioned into the wax rims (Figure 94).

There are four sizes of tracing plate and two sizes of stylus to choose from according to the size of the registration rims (Figure 95).

First warm the stylus over a Bunsen burner and seat onto the wax rim such that the stylus is over the midline in the premolar region. Similarly, heat the tracing plate onto the mandibular record block to be level with the occlusal plane. The mandibular plate can either be for taking the tracing only or the tracing can be carried out on the bite fork of a facebow.

Figure 93

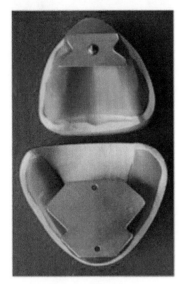

Figure 94

Adjustment of the tracing devices

With the rims in position, the patient is guided through lateral and protrusive excursions. If the rims touch, preventing a smooth movement, adjust the rim or increase the vertical dimension by unscrewing the stylus. This increase is closed down on the articulator in the laboratory once the models are mounted.

At this stage there should be no contact between the rims except between stylus and plate and you should ensure that the stylus does not slip behind the plate during protrusive excursions. If contact occurs, the vertical dimension should be increased or the rim adjusted. If the stylus slides off the plate, it should be moved further forward.

Wax crayon is applied to the plate and the patient is asked to make left and right lateral movements. Repeated movements – forwards and back, left and back, forwards and back, right and back – will need to be carried out to produce a clear tracing.

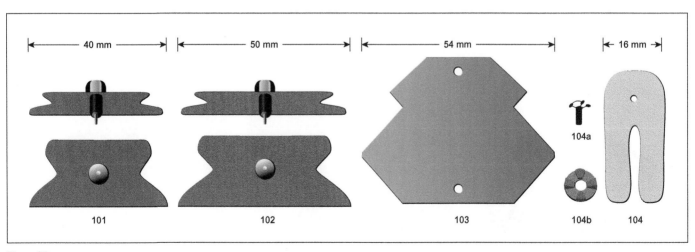

Figure 95

Some patients require a little practice to be able to carry out the movements easily, particularly those who have experienced occlusal problems with previous dentures, or who have excessive wear causing forward posturing. For those who find the movements hard to achieve, it can be more productive to ask them to move into as many different positions as possible; a clear tracing will eventually result. The tracing is usually a diamond shape, which is the full envelope of movement, the front apex of which is centric relation as shown in Figure 96.

Once a tracing has been made, a Perspex disc with a bevelled hole is positioned on the lower plate such that the centre of the hole is over the apex of the gothic arch tracing. It is fixed in position with sticky wax (Figure 97). Alternatively, if using a facebow a plastic holder may be screwed into place (Figure 98). In each case the diameter of the stylus is the same as that of the hole and the stylus should fit perfectly into the hole if the tracing has been performed correctly.

A 'V'-shaped notch is cut into either side of both wax blocks, where there is a recess in the mounting plates (Figure 99). This locates the rims together in RCP.

The registration rims are then replaced in the mouth and the patient encouraged to close together gently on the back teeth. With assistance, the mandible is positioned such that the stylus locates in the hole of the Perspex disc, as shown in Figure 91. Once the stylus has located into the hole, bite registration material is placed in the buccal corridors on both sides so that it reproduces the grooves made previously in the buccal surfaces of the wax blocks (Figure 92). Once set, the registration keys can be removed, along with the gothic arch tracing plates and used for mounting onto an articulator where the correct vertical dimension is re-established.

To avoid opening the vertical dimension at the recording stage, the upper rim may be reduced by 5 mm to accommodate the upper stylus (Figure 100). The correct occlusal dimension is re-established using the value measured previously between the wires by adjusting the stylus up or down by screwing or unscrewing as necessary.

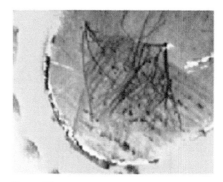

Figure 96

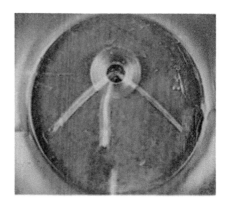

Figure 97

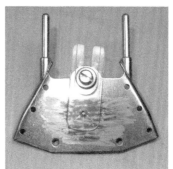

Figure 98

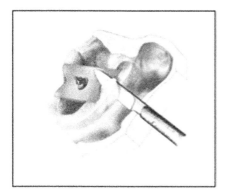

Figure 99

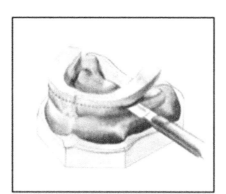

Figure 100

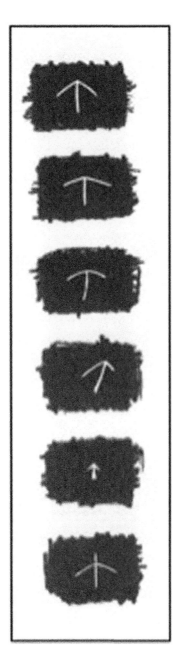

Figure 101

Evaluating different gothic arch tracings

Figure 101 shows some examples of the various forms of gothic arch tracings that may be seen and an explanation of their meaning is given below from top to bottom as you look at the tracings.

Classical pointed form: The symmetry indicates an undisturbed movement sequence in the joints and uniform muscle guidance.

Classical flat form: This indicates lateral movements of the condyles in the fossae.

Weak gothic arch tracing: This form indicates a lax and negligent performance of the movements. Repeat the registration.

Asymmetrical form: This indicates a distinct inhibition of the forward movement in the right joint.

Miniature gothic arch tracing: These cramp-like movements suggest a long edentulous state with inhibited movement in the joints.

Vertical line protrudes beyond the arrow point: This is caused by forcible retraction or pushing of the mandible, or may be obtained with a protruded mandible.

Chapter 5 | OCCLUSION, ARTICULATORS AND FACEBOWS

The occlusal schemes provided for complete dentures differ significantly from those found in most natural dentitions. The dentate occlusion is often canine guided or demonstrates group function. In each case the teeth contact on the working side but usually disclude on the non-working side in lateral excursions (Figure 102). Similarly, the posterior teeth disclude in protrusive excursions (Christensen's phenomenon) (Figure 103).

Dentures are different; the occlusion is designed to provide stability. Therefore the non-working side teeth also contact in lateral excursions to prevent the denture from tipping, giving rise to the term 'balancing side' (Figure 104a,b). The posterior teeth also contact in protrusive excursions as shown in Figure 105a,b for natural (a) and lingualised (b) teeth.

It can be a challenge to achieve such an occlusal scheme. The contacts must be harmonised in inter-cuspal position (ICP), lateral excursions and in the protrusive movement. To add to this challenge, the occlusal scheme must first be established on a device that mimics the patient's mandibular movements before being confirmed intraorally. It follows that the articulator on which the occlusal scheme is established should reproduce the movements of the mandible precisely, and allow for movements that may occur during mastication.

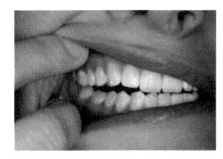

Figure 102

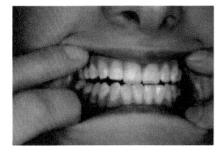

Figure 103

Balanced occlusion

Balanced occlusion refers to the occlusal scheme that is provided for dentures and features:

- inter-cuspal position (ICP) = retruded contact position (RCP);

- ICP on posterior teeth;

- working side and balancing side contacts in lateral excursions;

- anterior and posterior contact in protrusive excursions.

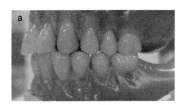

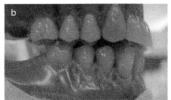

Figure 104

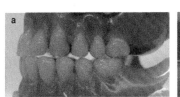 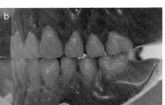

Figure 105

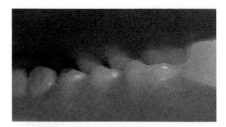

Figure 106

Inter-cuspal position = retruded contact position

The ICP contacts are established on the artificial teeth to coincide with the RCP position recorded at the registration stage. Having ICP and RCP coincident allows the wearer to function from centric relation, which is considered the optimal position for function and comfort.

Inter-cuspal position on posterior teeth

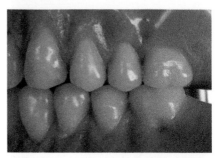

Figure 107

The ICP contacts are established between the palatal cusp of the upper teeth and the central fossae of the lower teeth, as shown in Figure 106. The buccal cusp of the lower also contacts the central fossae of the upper teeth (Figure 107).

ICP contacts may occur on anterior teeth where the skeletal classification permits (i.e. class III), which may be complicated by a crossbite (Figure 108).

Working side and balancing side contacts in lateral excursions

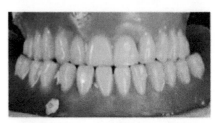

Figure 108

During excursions, the upper palatal cusps of the working side teeth maintain contact with the buccal facing slope of the lower lingual cusps as shown in Figure 109. The lower buccal cusp maintains contact with the palatal facing slope of the upper buccal cusp as shown in Figure 110.

On the balancing side, the upper palatal cusp maintains contact with the lingual facing slope of the buccal cusp as shown in Figure 111. The greater the number of balanced contacts during these excursions, the greater the stability of the denture.

Anterior and posterior contact in protrusive excursions

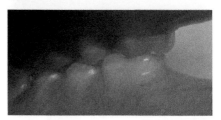

Figure 109

During protrusive excursions, the anterior teeth contact and simultaneous contact should be provided between the posterior teeth to prevent the dentures from dislodging (Figure 112). All of the contacts in excursions are produced to harmonise with the mandibular movement, which itself is determined by the movement of the condylar head as it travels down the articular eminence.

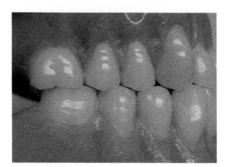

Figure 110

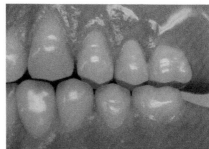

Figure 111

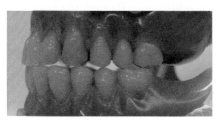

Figure 112

Lingualised occlusion

A modification of the balanced occlusion is the lingualised occlusion. This differs in that the artificial teeth are designed to have fewer ICP contacts (Figure 113a,b) while still distributing the occlusal load centrally over the alveolar ridge. In Figure 113 compare the lingualised occlusion teeth (patient left) with the natural occlusion teeth on the other side of the denture.

Similarly, when moved into lateral excursions, there is only one contact between the palatal cusp of the upper teeth and the buccal and lingual cusps of the lower teeth. To ensure the single contacts produce a stable denture, the occlusal contacts are positioned directly over the mandibular alveolar ridge, resulting in a narrower distribution of contacts and pressure, directed centrally over the ridges, compared to that seen when using natural occlusion teeth (Figure 114a,b).

This occlusal arrangement is also produced to conform to the mandibular movements of the mandible and thus also requires appropriate selection of articulator.

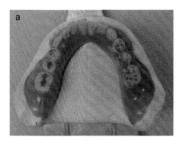
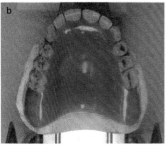

Figure 113

Types of articulator

There are four main types of articulator in use today:

- simple hinge;
- average value;
- semi adjustable;
- fully adjustable.

All articulators can hold models in ICP, however, this is the limitation of simple hinge articulators. Once the models are moved on the simple hinge articulator they travel on a different arc to that of the teeth in the mouth because the hinge is in the wrong place in comparison to the patient's temporomandibular joint. Therefore they do not replicate the opening movement of the mandible and cannot make lateral or protrusive excursions (Figure 115).

This problem also occurs in the 'Galetti', plasterless style articulator that has the condyle in an unrelated position to that of the patient, as shown in Figure 116.

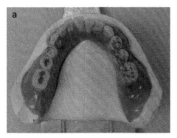
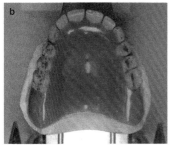

Figure 114

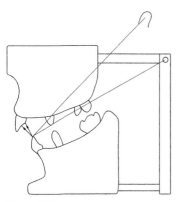

Figure 115

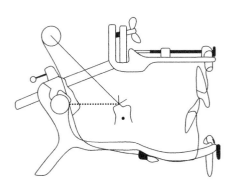

Figure 116

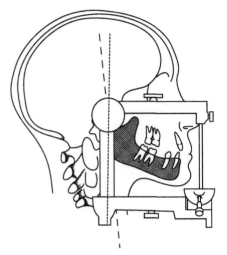

Figure 117

To duplicate the movement of the patient's mandible or teeth accurately, their relationship to the condyle must be duplicated on the articulator. This requires an anatomical articulator – either average value, semi-adjustable or fully adjustable – which is capable of replicating the anatomical arrangement (Figure 117).

Positioning the models correctly on the articulator allows them to be opened and closed in centric relation. It also allows adjustment of the vertical dimension while remaining in centric relation. Furthermore, positioning the models in the correct position allows movement into lateral excursions, as the movement hinges around the working side condylar head.

There are two methods of establishing the relationship between the models and the hinge. The first is to use an average value as determined by the Bonwill triangle; alternatively, the relationship between the teeth and the condyles (or maxilla, mandible and condyles for edentulous patients) can be recorded using a facebow.

When using a facebow the distance between the teeth and condyles is recorded mechanically and used to establish the position of the model on the articulator.

Although there are four main types of dental articulator, only three can be described as anatomical articulators. These can be categorised by their condylar guidance, giving rise to the three types: average value, semi-adjustable or fully adjustable.

Simple hinge articulators

This type of articulator only allows a hinge movement to be made and does not allow any lateral or protrusive excursions. It is therefore only of value when only the ICP is required to be observed (Figure 118a,b).

Average value articulators

This type of articulator has straight condylar paths that are set at 30°. The angle cannot be changed. The condylar path is flat, rather than curved like the natural condylar articular eminence (Figure 119).

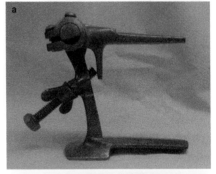

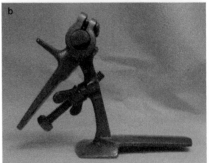

Figure 118

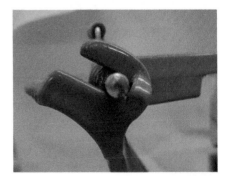

Figure 119

Semi-adjustable articulators

The majority of these articulators again have straight condylar paths, however the path angle may be changed, allowing the patient's condylar angle to be programmed into the articulator (Figure 120). This is still not a true representation of the articular eminence as it is a flat condylar pathway. Some semi-adjustable articulators have average value Bennett shift/movement built into the condylar head element, replicating the average head shape of the condyle (Figure 121a). This mimics the movement of the condyles better than some ball-shaped condylar heads found on other articulators (Figure 121b).

Fully adjustable articulators

These articulators attempt to go one step further; they allow the condylar paths to be adjusted such that the articulator mimics the movement of the condyle (Figure 122). The condylar movements are recorded using pantographic, stereographic or a computerised pantographic system. Figure 123 shows a Denar pantographic facebow used in conjunction with a fully adjustable articulator.

The recordings that are taken are replicated on the articulator by either adjusting the components of the articulator eminence on a fully adjustable articulator, or by reproducing the movements in self-curing acrylic. As shown in Figure 124, pantographic recordings can allow personalised incisal guidance tables to be created.

Intercondylar width

Some semi-adjustable articulators can be adjusted to take into account the differences that occur in intercondylar width. The width can be adjusted between 100 and 120 mm. The effect of adjusting this parameter has less effect on the pathway of the teeth or mandible than the adjustment of the condylar pathway. The effect of adjusting the intercondylar width can be seen in Figure 125. The pathway of the cusp is not affected in the functional range.

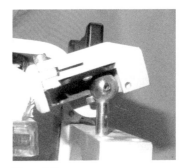

Figure 120

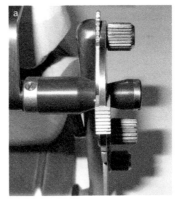

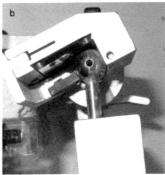

Figure 121

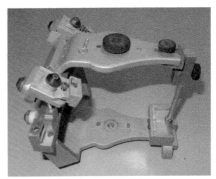

Figure 122

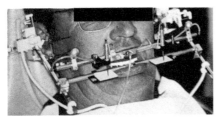

Figure 123

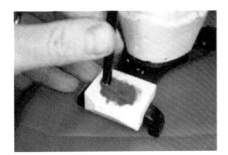

Figure 124

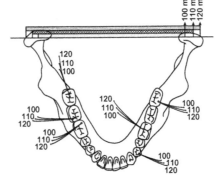

Figure 125

Bennett movement

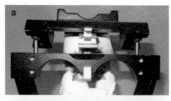
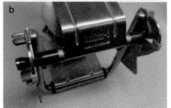

Figure 126

The ability to adjust the Bennett movement is also found on some semi-adjustable articulators. The Bennett movement is the lateral movement of the mandible as it moves towards the working side during excursions. The movement can be subdivided into immediate side shift and progressive side shift. The immediate side shift can take place in centric relation and can be considered as 'play' in the joint. The amount, up to 2.0 mm, can be measured and programmed into the articulator joint.

The medial wall of the non-working side temporomandibular joint (TMJ) determines progressive side shift. This determines the 'inward' component of the pathway that the condyle takes as it travels forwards and downwards in its non-working side movement. The average Bennett angle is 7°, but may be adjusted up to 15°. Other semi-adjustable articulators, such as the one shown in Figure 121a, have built-in Bennett movement.

'Arcon' or 'non-arcon'

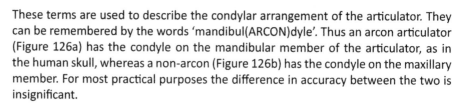

These terms are used to describe the condylar arrangement of the articulator. They can be remembered by the words 'mandibul(ARCON)dyle'. Thus an arcon articulator (Figure 126a) has the condyle on the mandibular member of the articulator, as in the human skull, whereas a non-arcon (Figure 126b) has the condyle on the maxillary member. For most practical purposes the difference in accuracy between the two is insignificant.

Denar articulators

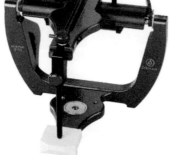

Figure 127

Denar produce a range of articulators designed for specific tasks:

Model 310

The Model 310 articulator shown in Figure 127 has been specifically designed for use with anterior guidance and posterior disclusion occlusal schemes. As such it has a protrusive condylar angle fixed at 25°, and progressive side shift fixed at 15°.

Comparable articulators are the Denar Automark and Whipmix Model 100.

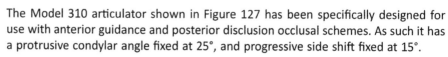

Model 320

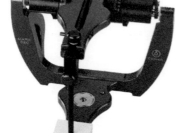

Figure 128

The Model 320 shown in Figure 128 allows the protrusive condylar angle to be adjusted, but has the fixed progressive side shift of 15°. This articulator is ideal when working with posterior disclusion of the non-working side with canine guidance or group function on the working side.

A comparable articulator is the Whipmix 2240.

Model 330

The Model 330 shown in Figure 129 allows the immediate and progressive side shift to be adjusted and therefore is ideal for use when working with a balanced occlusion.

Comparable articulators are the Ivoclar Stratos 200 and Ivoclar Stratos 300.

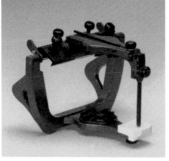

Figure 129

Condylator articulator

The Condylator articulator shown in Figure 130 is a semi-adjustable non-arcon design with a biconical axle that reproduces the anatomy of the condylar head. The Protrusive condylar pathway is adjustable but average values are used for intercondylar width and Bennett movement.

This articulator can be used for all types of restorative work, particularly complete and partial denture work.

Comparable articulators are the Candulor Articulator CAII, which accepts several different facebows.

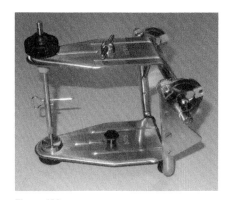
Figure 130

Types of facebow

Facebows can be used to:

- record the relationship between the condyles and the maxilla/mandible;
- record the incisal plane angle;
- determine the correct vertical position on the articulator;
- record the condylar angle (mandibular facebow); and
- record condylar movements (pantographic facebow).

Recording the relationship between the condyle and the maxilla/mandible

Facebows establish the relationship between the teeth and the condyles or in edentulous cases, between the maxilla/mandible and the condyles. Figure 131 shows four types of facebow: Dentatus facebow (Figure 131a), Denar facebow (Figure 131b), Condylator facebow (Figure 131c) and Denar pantagraphic facebow (Figure 131d).

Different designs of facebows record the relationship between either the mandible or the maxilla and the condyles. Maxillary facebows record the relationship between the maxillary teeth (or maxilla in edentulous cases) and condyles. Mandibular facebows record the relationship between the condyles and the mandibular teeth or mandible.

The facebow is used to position the respective model on the articulator so that the relationship between the patient's teeth (or edentulous ridges) and their condyle heads can be replicated on the articulator (Figure 132a,b).

A bite registration or registration rims, as shown in Figure 133, are used to mount the opposing model when a facebow has been used.

The facebow is more accurate and positions the models onto the articulator in the same relationship to the articulator's condylar elements as exist in the patient.

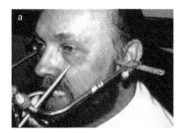
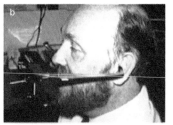
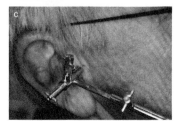
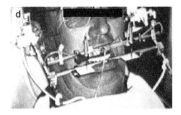
Figure 131

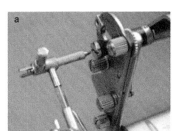
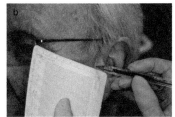
Figure 132

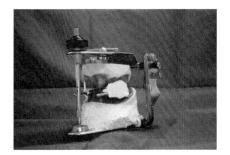
Figure 133

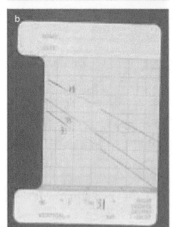

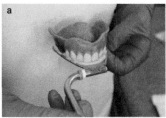

Figure 134

Recording the condylar angle

Mandibular facebows have the advantage that they allow the condylar angles to be recorded easily. Figure 134a shows a Condylator mandibular facebow being used to make condylar angle recordings (Figure 134b) which can then be transferred to the articulator.

When using a maxillary facebow, a separate procedure is necessary to record condylar angles.

Recording the incisal plane angle

Facebows help maintain the incisal plane angle. The facebow is aligned with the condyles and the eyes; this is then transferred to the articulator to mount the models in line with the articulator condyles.

Determining the correct vertical position on the articulator

Facebows also establish the vertical height of the models on the articulator. This ensures the condylar angle remains correct relative to the occlusal plane. A typical facebow procedure, using a Denar facebow, is shown in Figure 135a–d.

Recording condylar movements

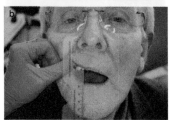

Pantographic facebows are used in conjunction with fully adjustable articulators to recreate the condylar pathway. They do this by recording both horizontal and vertical tracings of the condylar movement, as shown in Figure 131d.

Facebows may also differ in whether they use the actual condyle or an arbitrary position related to the condyle. Kinematic facebows locate the condyle precisely by positioning the arm of the facebow over the condyle (Figure 132a). As the mandible is open and closed on the terminal hinge axis; the arm rotates over the condyle. A pencil lead is incorporated to draw the result. The arm is adjusted until a single point tracing, rather than an arc tracing, is achieved. The facebow then uses this position to transfer the models to the articulator (Figure 132b).

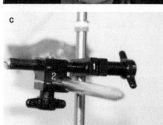

Arbitrarily positioned facebows have a method of locating the condyle built into the bow. For example, the Denar uses an earbow that is designed to compensate for the distance at which it sits behind the condyle (Figure 131d). These are often used because of their ease of operation.

Procedure for using a Denar facebow

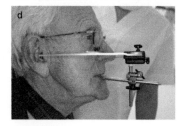

Figure 135

The Denar maxillary facebow records the relationship between the maxilla and condyles using an earbow. It also ensures that the incisal plane angle and the vertical height of the models on the articulator is correct. This facebow does not record condylar angle. To use the Denar facebow the following procedure is carried out at the occlusal registration stage once the vertical dimension has been established (here the anterior teeth have been positioned).

1. Attach the bite fork to the occlusal surface of the upper registration rim, ensuring that the bar exit is on the patient's right (Figure 135a).

2. Mark a reference position on the patient's face to establish the vertical position of the facebow (Figure 135b).

3. Secure the transfer jig in the earbow with the numbering facing you (Figure 135c).

4. With the screws loosened to allow free movement, slide the transfer jig onto the bite fork until the earbow is securely seated in the ear (Figure 135d).

5. Adjust the bow so that the vertical height indicator on the bow lines up with the reference position marked previously (Figure 136).

6. Tighten the screws on the transfer jig and check the bow to ensure that the registration rim is seated, the bow is in the ears and the height is correct.

7. The RCP record may now be taken and the facebow removed.

8. Next remove the transfer jig from the earbow ready for mounting the models on the articulator. Figure 137 shows the maxillary registration rim held in place on the bite folk with registration silicone.

9. Remove the incisal table from the articulator and replace with the articulating jig (Figure 138).

10. Position and secure the transfer jig onto the articulator (Figure 139).

11. The working cast may now be placed in the upper registration rim ready for plastering and secured if necessary (Figure 140). Care should be taken to ensure that the weight of the model does not cause movement of the transfer jig. Sometimes the weight of the model can bend the bite fork. If necessary, the device shown in Figure 141 can be attached to the mandibular arm of the articulator and adjusted to support the bite fork and prevent distortion when the model is attached.

12. Next, mount the maxillary model to the articulator (Figure 142).

13. Then attach the mandibular model using the RCP record (Figure 143a,b).

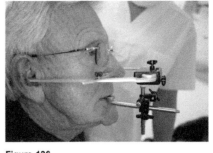

Figure 136

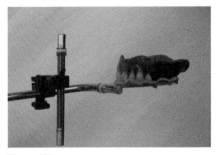

Figure 137

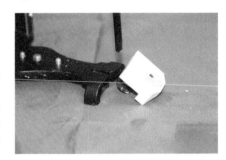

Figure 138

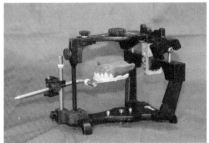

Figure 139

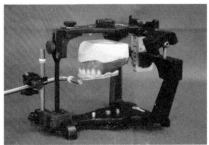

Figure 140

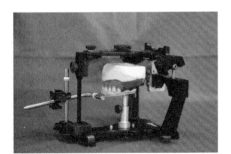

Figure 141

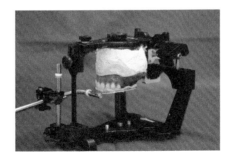

Figure 142

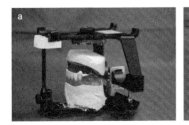

Figure 143

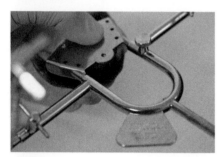

Figure 144

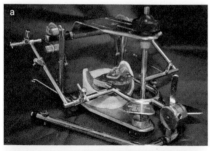

Figure 145

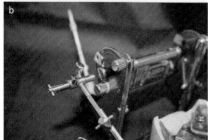

Figure 146

Procedure for using a Condylator facebow

The Condylator mandibular facebow can be used to establish and record the relationship between the mandible and condyle, and record the condylar angle. It is often used in conjunction with gothic arch tracing to record centric relation.

The following procedure is carried out at the occlusal registration stage once the vertical dimension has been established.

1. Select an appropriately sized biteplate and attach to the occlusal surface of the lower registration rim, ensuring that the surface is flush with the occlusal plane (Figure 144).

2. Mark a reference position over the patient's condyle, either by palpating for the condyle or measuring 13 mm anteriorly from the tragus of the ear on a line between the tragus and the outer canthus of the eye (ala-tragal or Camper's line) (see Figure 132b).

3. Position the bow on the biteplate (Figure 145). Then place the registration rim into the patient's mouth and adjust the facebow to fit around the face.

4. With the screws loosened to allow free movement, position and secure the arms of the facebow with the stylus over the condyles (see Figure 131c).

5. The facebow can now be removed and the centric relation (CR) record taken.

6. Next, secure the working model to the lower rim.

7. Position the facebow around the articulator such that the sprung writing point holders align with the centre of the condyles using the universal adjustment nut on the stand. This replicates the position recorded on the patient (Figure 146a,b).

8. Secure the lower model to the articulator and mount the upper using the CR record (Figure 147).

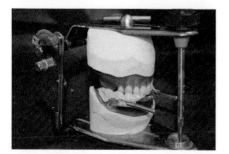

Figure 147

Split cast mounting technique

This technique is a simple method allowing the models to be mounted onto the articulator and then removed and replaced back onto the mounting plaster at will (Figure 148a,b). Steep chamfered cuts are made down the side of the models using a model trimmer (Figure 149a,b). The chamfered sections and the bottom of the model are then coated in plaster separating medium prior to the mounting plaster being applied. Once the mounting plaster is set and trimmed, the model can be detached from the mounting plaster by sharply tapping the join line between model and plaster.

To reattach the model to the mounting plaster the model is accurately positioned into the mounting plaster and model cement (sticky wax) is run along the junction between the two (Figure 150a,b).

Recording the condylar angle in conjunction with gothic arch tracing using a Gerber facebow

The GAT devices described here can be used without a facebow. Well-constructed, correctly extended registration rims are essential for stability when carrying out this procedure, which is carried out at the occlusal registration stage once the vertical dimension has been established.

During this procedure, the vertical dimension is lost when the GAT is carried out. Therefore before starting a piece of wire is inserted into the labial surface of each rim and the vertical dimension recorded using a pair of dividers as shown in Figure 151. The distance between these points is re-established once the stylus and plate have been positioned into the wax rims.

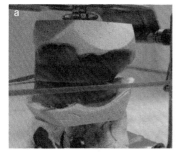
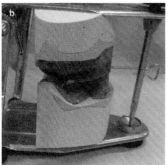

Figure 148

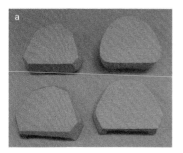
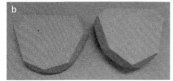

Figure 149

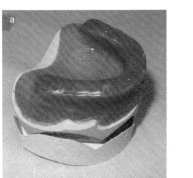
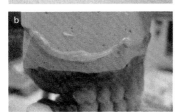

Figure 150

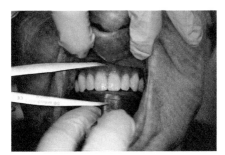

Figure 151

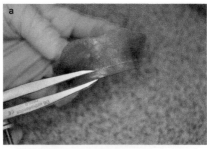

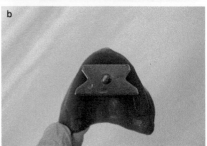

Figure 152

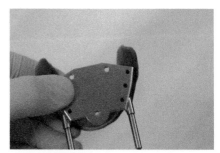

Figure 153

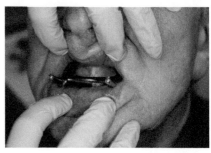

Figure 154

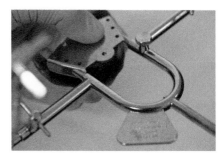

Figure 155

1. Mark a reference position over the patient's condyle, either by palpating for the condyle or measuring 13 mm anteriorly to the tragus of the ear on a line between the tragus and the outer canthus of the eye (see Figure 132b).

2. Select a tracing plate and stylus. There are four sizes of tracing plate and two sizes of stylus to choose from according to the size of the registration rims (see Figure 144).

3. Remove 5 mm of wax from the maxillary rim (Figure 152a).

4. Warm the stylus over a Bunsen burner and seat onto the wax rim such that the stylus is over the midline in the premolar region (Figure 152b).

5. Choose a lower biteplate to fit the mandibular registration block and secure it using sticky wax (Figure 153).

6. Place the registration rims are placed in the mouth and check to ensure that the stylus contacts the lower plate with no other contacts.

7. The face height can now be adjusted using the stylus to the measure previously recorded between the pieces of wire (Figure 154).

8. Guide the patient through lateral and protrusive excursions. At this stage there should be no contact between the rims except between stylus and plate. Ensure that the stylus does not slip behind the plate during protrusion. If contact occurs, the vertical dimension should be increased or the rim adjusted. If the stylus slides off the plate, it should be moved further forward.

9. With the facebow tipped towards the operator, position the bow on the biteplate (Figure 155). Ask the patient to close together to prevent tipping of the facebow.

10. With the screws loosened to allow free movement, position the arms of the facebow with the stylus over the condyles and secure them. The housing for the spring loaded pencil should be approximately 1 mm away from the skin (Figure 156).

11. Once the patient has practised protrusive and retrusive movements, and can do so on request, place a tracing card between the skin and pencil housing.

12. Orientate the card so that the horizontal lines are parallel to the horizontal occlusal plane indicator arm on the facebow.

13. Hold the card securely from behind the patient to ensure that it remains stable during movement.

14. With the patient in the retruded position, gently release the pencil onto the card and instruct the patient to make protrusive movements of the mandible (Figure 157).

15. Remove the pencil from the card. This procedure is carried out three times on each side to ensure the tracings are consistent.

16. Next, remove the facebow from the registration rims and secure it to its stand using the universal joint. Make sure all joints are securely fastened before storing or using the facebow to mount the models.

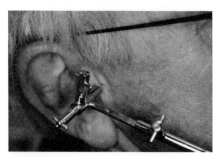

Figure 156

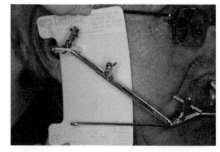

Figure 157

The gothic arch tracing is now carried out to establish centric relation. Wax crayon or 'engineer's blue' is applied to the biteplate and the patient is asked to make left and right lateral and protrusive movements. Repeated movements – forwards and back, left and back, forwards and back, right and back – will need to be carried out to produce a clear tracing (Figure 158).

Some patients require a little practice to be able to carry out the movements easily, particularly those whose previous dentures were not made to centric relation or have excessive wear, causing forward posturing.

For those who find the movements hard to achieve, it can be more productive to ask them to move into as many different positions as possible, a clear tracing will eventually result. The tracing is usually a diamond shape, as shown in Figure 159. The CR position is the anterior apex.

Once a tracing has been made, a Perspex disc with a bevelled hole is positioned on the lower plate such that the centre of the hole is over the apex of the gothic arch tracing. It is fixed in position with sticky wax or model cement as shown in Figure 160. The stylus diameter is the same as the diameter of the hole in the disc so the stylus should fit perfectly into the hole if the tracing has been performed correctly (Figure 161). The position is recorded using impression plaster or silicone bite registration material (Figure 162).

Transferring the condylar angle recordings to the articulator

Tangents drawn through the condylar angle tracings can be measured using a protractor, using an average of three tracings per condyle. This angle can then be transferred to the articulator (Figure 163a,b).

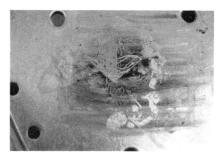

Figure 158

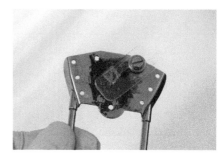

Figure 159

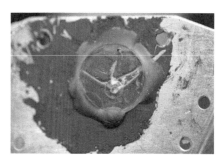

Figure 160

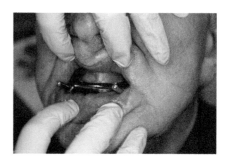

Figure 161

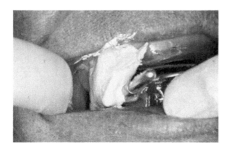

Figure 162

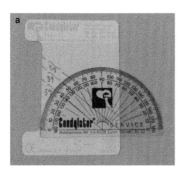
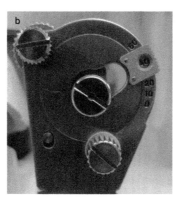

Figure 163

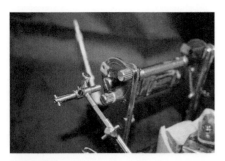

Figure 164

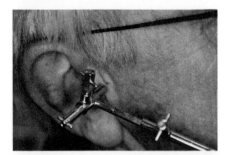

Figure 165

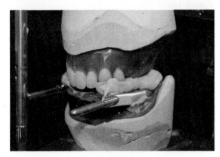

Figure 166

The facebow is used to mount the lower model on the articulator. The position is adjusted using the universal joint on the stand, so that the pencil leads are pointing into the centres of the condyle head of the articulator (Figure 164). This replicates the relationship of the facebow when it was attached to the patient as shown in Figure 165.

The mandibular model is attached to the bite fork using sticky wax and attached to the lower arm of the articulator using plaster of Paris and the maxillary registration rim and model are related to the mandibular model using the plaster or silicone bite registrations (Figure 166).

Sometimes the procedure can be carried out without having to reduce the maxillary rim by carrying out the recordings at an increased vertical dimension. This means that the condyle path tracings will be inclined 4–6° more horizontally and the vertical dimension of the articulator should be increased prior to mounting the upper model.

This method also has an effect on the condylar inclination recording, so this should be compensated for by adding one half degree (or 30 angular minutes) to the condyle path angle for each millimetre increase in the vertical dimension measured at the vertical pin of the Condylator articulator.

Chapter 6 | AESTHETICS

The occlusal registration stage should incorporate the positioning of the anterior teeth or at least the selection of size, shape and shade. This chapter discusses how to select the appropriate teeth and how these should be arranged.

Duplicating aesthetics

The most reliable method of achieving the desired appearance is to copy the arrangement of the patient's natural teeth or that from a previous denture, if liked by the patient.

Natural teeth

Pictures of natural teeth are enormously useful in determining the shape and size of the teeth that should be used. The appropriate mould can be selected and aged by creating wear and staining, if required (this is more usually applied with partial dentures when matching denture teeth next to natural teeth), to create an approximation of the patient's natural teeth.

From the picture of a patient showing their teeth it is possible to estimate the size of the teeth by using the following calculations.

1. Measure the inter-pupillary distance on the patient.

2. Divide this by the inter-pupillary distance on the photograph.

3. Multiply this by the width of the two incisor teeth on the photograph.

4. Divide this by 2 to give the width of one central incisor.

This measurement of the central incisor width can then be used to select the correct width of teeth required from the appropriate mould chart, which usually has the width of the central incisors for all the teeth indicated.

Existing dentures

Having an impression of the existing dentures allows the technician to easily copy any features of the existing dentures that are to be retained. Photographs of the patient wearing their dentures can also be useful in establishing shortfalls or positive aspects about the dentures' appearance.

Techniques in Complete Denture Technology, First Edition. Tony Johnson, Duncan J. Wood.
© 2012 Tony Johnson and Duncan J. Wood. Published 2012 by Blackwell Publishing Ltd.

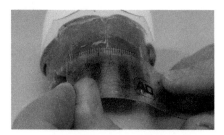

Figure 167

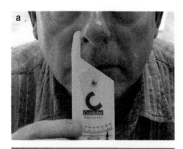

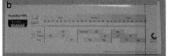

Figure 168

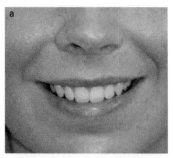

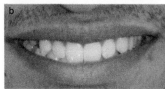

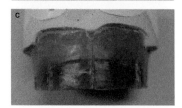

Figure 169

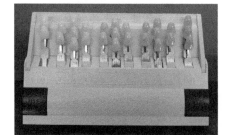

Figure 170

Selecting denture teeth

Size

To establish the overall width of the six anterior teeth, the distance between the canines can be determined using various methods:

- Marking the corners of the mouth on the rim with the mouth at rest. A measurement can now be taken directly from the rim as shown in Figure 167.

- Using a straight edge aligned with the inner canthus of the eye and the ala of the nose to find the position of the canine. Again this is marked directly on to the rim.

- Measuring the width of the nose at its widest point with the mouth at rest. Add 5 mm to this measurement to allow for the curvature of the teeth.

- Using an Alameter, supplied by Candulor, to give an estimate of the tooth size required by using the maximum width of the nose. This device suggests the mould numbers from the Candulor range that would be most appropriate (Figure 168a,b).

The width of the two central incisors may be estimated using the philtrum width as shown in Figure 169a. The height of the central incisor should be equal to or greater than the height of the smile line above the incisal edge (Figure 169b). This high smile line should ideally be marked onto the wax rim of the registration rim during the registration stage by the clinician (Figure 169c).

Larger central incisors should be used for people with a high lip line, those of large stature and those with large faces.

Shade

Colour is described using the terms 'value' (lightness), 'chroma' (saturation) and 'hue' (colour), as shown on the Vita 3D-Master shade guide illustrated in Figure 170.

The lightness (value) of the tooth should first be selected to harmonise with the patient's complexion. In general, darker teeth should be selected for older patients. Figure 171a shows an elderly patient with denture teeth that are too light in colour for his age and skin tone. A more suitable shade of tooth has been selected in Figure 171b.

Once the lightness has been selected, the colour saturation (chroma) should be chosen. This property can be varied between the teeth to give a natural appearance. For example, if a darker canine is required, the next available chroma may be selected.

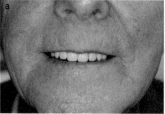
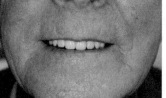
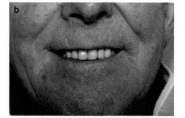

Figure 171

The colour of the tooth (hue) should then be chosen; this is the property to which the human eye is least sensitive.

The classic shade guide can also be used by rearranging the shade tabs using the following protocol.

1. Determine the lightness value or level:

   - Hold the shade guide to the patient's mouth at arms length.

   - Select from groups 1, 2, 3, 4 or 5 (Figure 172a).

   - Start your selection with the darkest group first and select the most appropriate tab to match the patient's skin tone.

2. Select the chroma:

   - Using the lightness level chosen, take out the middle hue group (M) and spread the sample out like a fan (Figure 172b,c).

   - Select the one of the three shade samples that matches best.

3. Determine the hue:

   - Check whether the teeth required should be more reddish or more yellowish than the shade sample selected by replacing the M group tab and looking either side of this at the L and R tabs (Figure 172d).

Other tooth manufacturers' shade guides may not be as comprehensive as the Vita 3D-Master but should be used using the same principles.

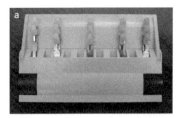
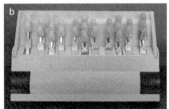
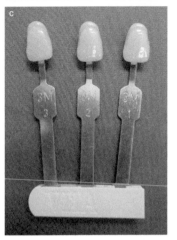
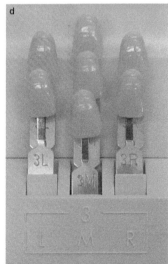

Figure 172

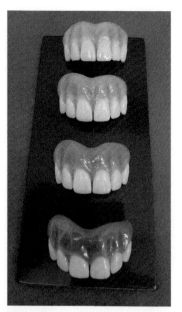

Figure 173

There are many different shades of polymethyl methacrylate (PMMA) available on the market to suit every ethnic skin tone. Different shades of PMMA can have a dramatic effect on the chosen tooth shade (Figure 173). PMMA shade guides are available from good manufacturers (Figure 174), although they are very rarely used in general practice.

Shape

Teeth moulds are available for patients with round, square or tapering faces. Each is available in a range of sizes.

Several methods have been described for selecting tooth shape:

- Use the patient's old dentures if they are happy with the teeth.

- Select teeth based on the inverted shape of the patient's face to determine whether the teeth should be square, tapering, ovoid or oblong (Figure 175).

- Select teeth based on the shape of the patient's upper palate (Figure 175).

Masculine and feminine moulds are always available for selection (Figure 176).

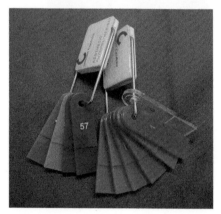

Figure 174

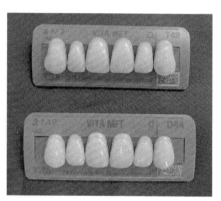

Figure 176

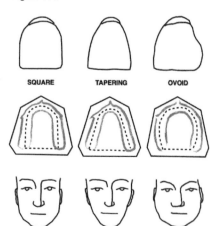

SQUARE   TAPERING   OVOID

Figure 175

Where no record of the patient's natural teeth is available, the patient's facial features can be used to aid the selection of shape and arrangement of teeth. Look at the shape of the patient's face and decide which of the four mould types complements their features.

- Square teeth (Figure 177a,b) complement a square set face and strong features.

- Ovoid teeth (Figure 178a,b) create 'softer' appearance and complement delicate, rounded features.

- Tapering teeth (Figure 179a,b) best suit the tapering face shape.

- Rectangular teeth (Figure 180a,b) suit the 'long square' shaped face best. (It should be noted that not all tooth manufacturers' produce and a rectangular mould of tooth.)

Tooth arrangement

The arrangement of the teeth is also a decision that should be made with the patient. Useful questions to ask include the following.

- Should the new denture teeth replicate the old dentures?

- Should they be a 'standard' arrangement?

- Should they be arranged to copy the patient's natural teeth (here a photograph of the patient with teeth would be needed and the teeth aged as if natural wear had taken place)?

A joint decision with the patient at this stage can save a lot of time later.

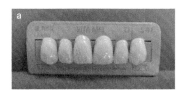
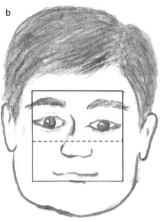

Figure 177

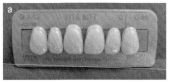
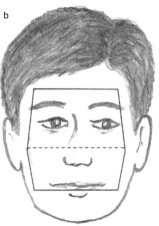

Figure 178

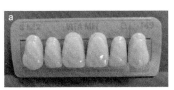
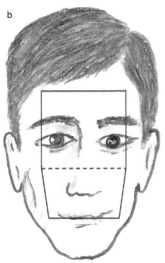

Figure 179

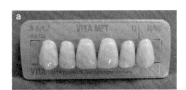
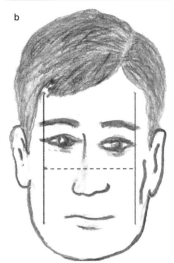

Figure 180

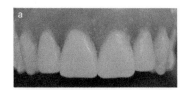
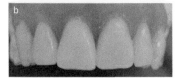
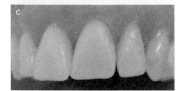

Figure 181

Positioning anterior teeth

It is very often difficult to 'personalise' denture teeth to an individual patient. Modification of the 'basic or standardised NHS type' dental arch arrangement, as shown in Figure 181, to reflect outstanding facial characteristics of the individual patient can be one way to achieve this. Figure 181a shows a typical 'NHS' arrangement of maxillary anterior denture teeth. The teeth are usually positioned to be identical on both sides, which is a situation very rarely seen in nature. Figures 181b,c show the same teeth with subtle differences between the right and left sides and with small diastemas and embrasures built into the arrangement to try to replicate what we normally see in the natural condition. Slight differences in the angles of left and right sided teeth and in the lengths of teeth can create a more natural appearance.

Other tips to achieve a natural look include the following.

- Ensure that the incisal plane is made parallel to the lip line. In Figure 182 the occlusal plane of the maxillary anterior teeth conforms to the shape of the lower lip when the patient is smiling.

- Align the long axis of the central incisors with the philtrum (Figure 183).

- A more masculine appearance can be created by making a reverse curve on the centrals (have the distal aspects placed more anteriorly than the mesial aspects). This will make them appear wider to match the forehead-widening effects of horizontal eyebrows (Figure 184).

- Conversely, having the laterals slightly forward of the centrals (class II division II ish) and rotating the centrals distally to make them appear narrower will match the forehead-narrowing effect of highly angular eyebrows and create a more feminine appearance (Figure 185).

- Laterals and canines can be rotated mesially to make them appear wider to match the widening effects of flattened cheeks for both horizontal and angular eyebrows.

- Laterals and canines can be rotated distally to make them appear narrower to match the narrowing effects of receding cheeks for both horizontal and angular eyebrows (Figure 186).

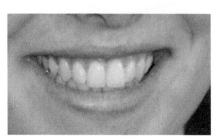

Figure 182

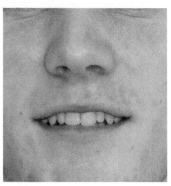

Figure 183

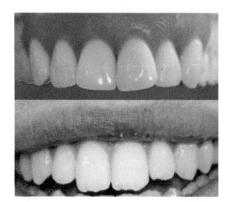

Figure 184

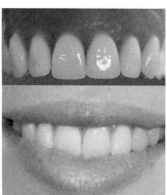

Figure 185

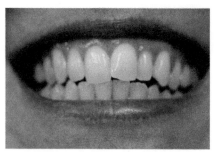

Figure 186

- The angles of the labial surface of the centrals and lateral incisors can be arranged such that they conform to a line drawn from the angle of the forehead at the top of the nose down through the base of the nose and on to just touch the tip of the chin (Figure 187).

- The central and lateral incisors can be positioned to follow any deviation of the nose from the midline (Figure 188).

- The angle of the canine should be made to harmonise with the angle of the cheeks. (Figure 189).

- The lower incisors should be placed to create a natural angle for the lower lip (Figure 190). The actual position of the lower incisors can be controlled by the clinician using a modified neutral zone technique, which records the position, and to some extent the angle, of the lip when it is in its most extended position (Figure 191).

- Many technicians and dentists tend to concentrate on the maxillary teeth as far as aesthetics is concerned. The mandibular anterior teeth are just as important, and are very often seen more than the maxillary teeth in older patients. Asymmetrical setting of the teeth looks more natural (Figure 192). Making subtle changes in tooth angle and spacing between the right and left anterior teeth to complement the 'strong' side of the face can create a more natural appearance.

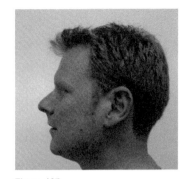

Figure 187

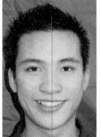 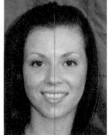

Figure 188

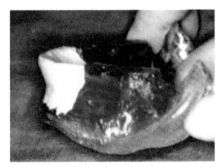

Figure 191

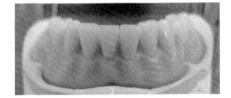

Figure 192

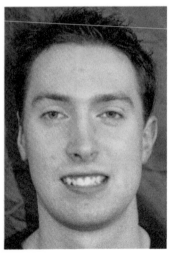

Figure 189

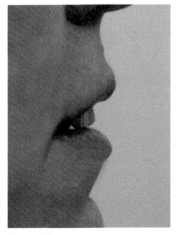

Figure 190

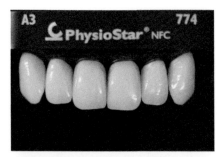

Figure 193

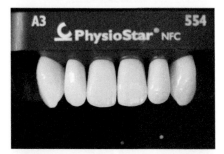

Figure 194

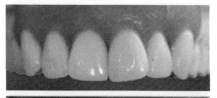

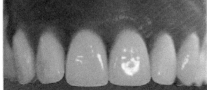

Figure 195

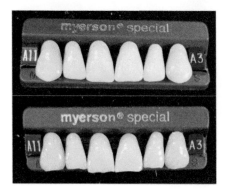

Figure 196

Masculine and feminine

In general, squarer, well-defined teeth create a masculine appearance, where subtler or more rounded tooth moulds are selected to create a feminine appearance. Figure 193 shows a typically masculine looking set of teeth, whereas Figure 194 shows a typically feminine looking set of teeth.

Even using the same tooth mould, the teeth may be arranged to create a harsher or softer look, as illustrated in Figure 195.

Changing the shape of teeth

Where teeth have been selected and the size or shape is slightly wrong, the teeth can be reshaped using a tungsten bur and silicone polishing bur. Often only the labial surface and incisal edge need be adjusted to create a different tooth shape, without the need for trimming the mesial and distal surfaces. Most artificial tooth manufacturers produce anterior teeth with perfect incisal edges with lovely translucent tips! The majority of denture wearers, being elderly, would not naturally have perfect, translucently tipped anterior teeth. Leaving the teeth in this 'perfect' state, as shown in Figure 196 (top), would look unnatural, and on an older patient's dentures a more natural effect can be created by adding a good degree of incisal edge wear, as shown in Figure 196 (bottom).

Similarly, the shape of a tooth can be 'changed' by adjusting the gingival contour. Here the tooth mould and arrangement is the same, but shaping the gingival margin alters the outline of the tooth (Figure 197).

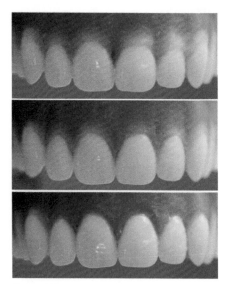

Figure 197

Characterising teeth

Colour of canines

One of the most simple yet effective characterisations is to change the colour of the canine teeth and break-up uniformity of the denture. Canines are always significantly darker in the natural dentition and copying this natural feature improves the appearance of dentures hugely. Having the canines half to one shade darker than the centrals and incisor teeth as shown in Figure 198a,b will replicate the natural condition.

The anterior denture teeth are usually supplied together, however some manufacturers will sell individual pairs to allow darker canines to be placed (Figure 199).

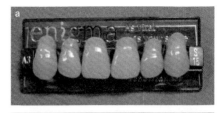
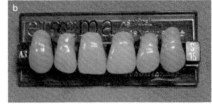

Figure 198

Providing wear

Most denture wearers tend to be elderly and would have worn down their natural teeth if they still had any. It is therefore reasonable to expect the wear on their denture teeth to reflect the natural wear if natural aesthetics are to be achieved. The teeth will benefit from having the appropriate amount of wear such that they look as if wearing over each other has shaped them.

Natural teeth wear in several ways. First, wear facets develop through attrition as opposing teeth occlude, as shown in Figure 200. This type of wear is best recreated at the 'grinding-in stage', after the dentures have been processed. During lateral and protrusive excursions the antagonistic contacts can be ground to effectively simulate the amount of wear that would be expected of someone of the patient's age. In Figure 200 the natural tooth wear situation is seen and in Figure 201 it is replicated in the denture teeth.

To replicate wear characteristics, first look for the areas of the teeth that contact in excursions. Then holding the bur parallel to the direction of the movement, reduce the incisal edge to allow greater contact of the teeth. Repeat until the desired effect is achieved (Figure 202a,b). This process will also remove the translucent enamel area of the tooth, which again mimics the appearance of the older natural tooth where required.

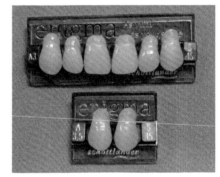

Figure 199

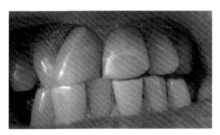

Figure 200

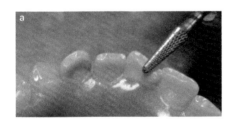
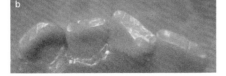

Figure 202

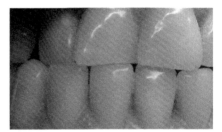

Figure 201

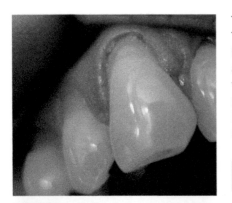

Figure 203

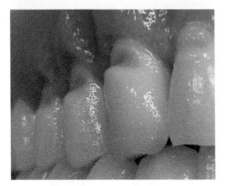

Figure 204

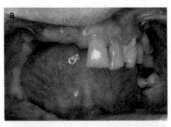

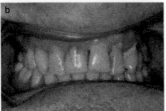

Figure 205

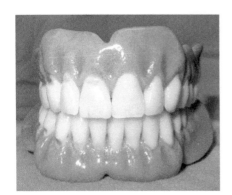

Figure 206

Teeth also wear through abrasion where an abrasive has worn away tooth material. The most common cause of this is the abrasive property of toothpaste on toothbrush. This removes tooth material evenly over the whole tooth surface and may also create deeper abrasion cavities towards the gingival margin. Replicating this wear pattern can be particularly effective if carried out on the canine and first premolar teeth. Staining the cervical area of the tooth may also enhance this feature. Figure 203 shows abrasion cavities and staining on natural teeth and Figure 204 shows cavities and staining recreated on denture teeth.

Staining teeth

Characterising the teeth using stains is most useful where natural, heavily stained teeth remain and a colour match is required (Figure 205a,b). Staining of individual teeth can help to disguise a complete denture, particularly in conjunction with wear facets. The left hand side of the complete denture case shown in Figure 206 has been characterised to show the effects that can be created, if necessary.

Tooth staining kits are available for resin or porcelain teeth in a range of colours (Figure 207).

Dealing with high lip and smile lines

In these situations it is not possible to 'fill' the entire smile with teeth as the result would be unnatural with long teeth. The best solution is to use a tooth mould that helps fill the smile, but to concentrate on creating a natural gingival contour.

First, the shape of the gingival margin should be produced to reveal the necks of the teeth. The wax is symmetrically carved around the teeth to create gingival margins that match the age of the patient as shown in Figure 208.

Interproximally, the wax should be reduced to create shadowing between the teeth, which helps to emphasise the colour of the gingivae. In Figure 209 the finished waxwork shows symmetrically shaped gingival margins and root eminences creating shadowing between the teeth which helps to replicate the natural condition.

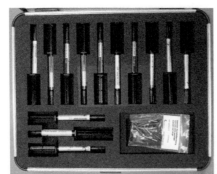

Figure 207

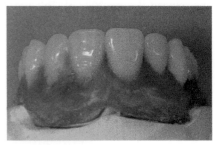

Figure 208

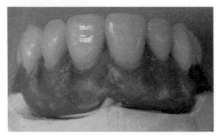

Figure 209

Stippling should be used to create a surface finish that scatters the light falling on the surface. In Figure 210 light stippling of the labial surfaces helps to defuse and scatter the light entering the mouth and creates a more natural appearance, helping the acrylic material to blend into the surrounding tissues.

Gingival staining can also be carried out to create subtle changes in colour around the teeth. Figure 211 shows an example of an upper ethnic resin denture stained to match the gingival colour of the natural lower dentition for an Afro-Caribbean patient.

Denture teeth

There are numerous ranges of teeth available from a number of manufacturers. The main criteria for selection of anterior teeth are aesthetics, although the material type – acrylic, composite or porcelain – is sometimes a consideration.

Acrylic teeth have advanced significantly in recent years and are often made from highly cross-linked acrylic that improves wear resistance and colour stability. The more advanced teeth are produced from numerous layers of different coloured acrylic, resulting in excellent aesthetic properties.

Composites are generally harder and longer lasting than acrylic, and have superb aesthetic properties, although one disadvantage is the reduced bond strength to the underlying acrylic. Many of these teeth have an acrylic 'core' which can sometimes be ground thin or even ground away completely when fitting the teeth. This may be resolved by providing mechanical retention to the underside of the teeth.

Porcelain teeth are less common but are available. The retention to the denture base is achieved through mechanical features called diatoric holes designed into the teeth.

In Figure 212 a comparison is shown between identical shades and moulds of acrylic (left), composite (middle) and porcelain (right) denture teeth. The top panel in Figure 212 shows the teeth back lit and the bottom panel shows them lit from the front.

When selecting posterior teeth, the type of occlusal arrangement should be the principal factor. Teeth are available to suit conventional balanced occlusion, lingualised occlusion, or with relatively flat occlusal surfaces for those with functional problems.

A range of denture teeth by leading manufacturers is presented and described below.

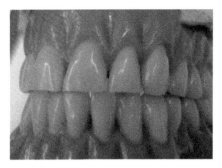

Figure 210

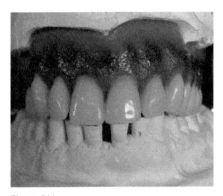

Figure 211

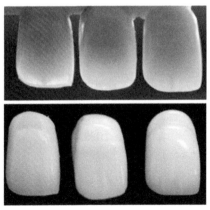

Figure 212

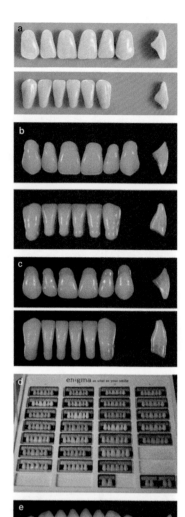

Figure 213

Schottlander

Delphic (acrylic)

These are Schottlander's entry-level teeth. They are available in an extensive range of 18 upper anterior moulds and 8 lower anterior moulds. The shade range includes sixteen A1–D4 shades as well as additional 'O' and 'G' shade ranges for greater warmth and graduated grey shades, respectively.

The posterior tooth moulds are available in three types: Traditional, Easy-set and Perfection. The Perfection range has 'freely interacting cusps', allowing quick setting and stability in the mouth. They are also narrower bucco-lingually. The Easy-set teeth (Figure 213a) have more pronounced cusp angles.

Natura

Schottlander's mid-range tooth, Natura (Figure 213b), includes internal mamelon effects and opalescence to improve aesthetics over the Delphic range. The 19 anterior moulds are grouped into tapered, square and oval moulds with a good range of sizes in each. The lower anterior moulds are available in seven sizes and also include the aesthetic features. The anteriors are supported by five posterior mould sizes that also have translucent cusps for improved aesthetics.

Enigma

This is Schottlander's flagship range produced from a double cross-linked acrylic, resulting in teeth which are harder and more colour stable than regular teeth (Figure 213c). The teeth are produced from multiple layers of acrylic, resulting in a vibrant-looking tooth, and they incorporate features such as internal mamelons, darker and longer necks, darker canine teeth, demineralisation points and opalescence of the material.

The range consists of 27 anterior moulds, again divided into oval, square and tapering groups. There are two groups of tapering, the second featuring teeth laterals with greater height to width ratios (Figure 213d). The teeth are also available to purchase in pairs, allowing for the mixing of shades at no extra cost. The shade range extends from A1 to D4 with additional bleaching shades.

The posterior teeth have 23° cusp angles and well-defined occlusal contact points. The tooth design also includes reduced lingual cusps in order to increase tongue space. Typical Enigma posterior teeth can be seen in Figure 213e.

Candulor

Preference (PMMA)

This is Candulor's entry-level tooth, made of triple-layered PMMA and available in the Vita Classic shades and two bleaching shades. Five sizes of anterior oval, triangular and square moulds make up the range with five lower anterior sizes to correspond. The posterior teeth are available in three sizes and have a multifunctional design of occlusal surface.

PhysioSet TCR (twin cross-linked)

These cross-linked PMMA resin teeth are multilayered for improved aesthetics and have more pronounced surface contours (Figure 214a). As shown in Figure 214c, the range comprises 22 upper anterior moulds, again divided into oval, triangular and square, which combine with a choice of five Bonartic posterior moulds (Figure 214b).

PhysioStar NFC (nano-filled composite)

These teeth are produced from two layers of composite, which provide excellent aesthetics and wear resistance, and two layers of PMMA to provide bonding to the acrylic (Figure 214d). As shown in Figure 214e, the range consists of 15 upper anterior moulds divided into four groups: Delicate, Universal, Vigorous and Individual. These combine with four lower anterior moulds.

These anterior teeth combine with either Condyloform II NFC (Figure 214f) or Bonartic NFC (Figure 214g) posterior moulds, which again offer improved wear resistance and colour stability, and are available in three sizes. The Condyloform II teeth are ideal for lingualised occlusion arrangements.

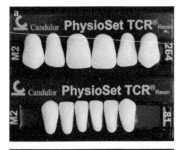
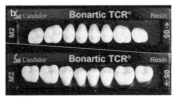
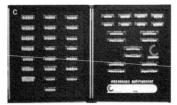
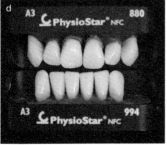
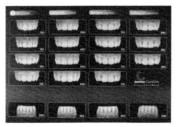
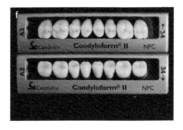
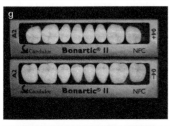
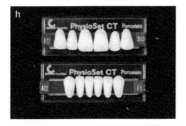
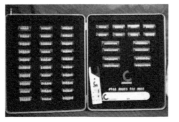
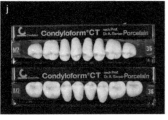
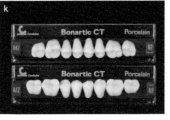

Figure 214

PhysioSet CT (porcelain)

These teeth (Figure 214h) are produced from six layers of porcelain, resulting in a tooth with a natural appearance with translucency and vitality. Being porcelain they also have high abrasion resistance and colour stability. The teeth are retained in the acrylic base by either a metal pin or a hole in the ceramic to create mechanical retention. As shown in Figure 214i, the range consists of 30 upper anterior moulds and 8 lower anterior moulds, available in the Candulor shade range. The moulds are again grouped as oval, triangular or square.

The porcelain range has two types of posterior teeth, Condyloform CT (Figure 214j) for lingualised occlusion available in five sizes, or Bonartic CT Porcelain (Figure 214k) available in four sizes.

Candulor supply a guide to selecting the correct tooth size from the TCR, NFC or CT range. The width of the nose is measured and, using the guide, the most appropriately sized teeth may be determined.

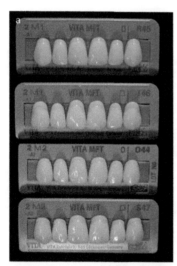

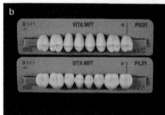

Figure 215

Vita

Vita MFT (multifunctional teeth) acrylic teeth

This is Vita's 'economy' range, although the aesthetic quality is good as a result of being produced from three layers of different coloured acrylic (Figure 215a). It is available in a limited range of eight of the most popular 3D-Master/Classic shades, with 12 upper anterior and 5 lower anterior. However, the mould range is simple and logical, with O, T, R and S for ovoid, triangular, rectangular and square, respectively, and the sizes of the six anterior teeth follow the letter.

The posteriors are designed to allow conventional or ligualised occlusion with 20° cusp angles. The lowers are 'abraded' for a little more flexibility and available in three sizes: 29, 31 and 33 mm (Figure 215b).

Vitapan: acrylic teeth

Vita's mid-range tooth includes aesthetic features such as enamel cracks, calcification marks and dentine clouds. It is available in 26 3D-Master shades as well as the 15 Vita Classical shades. The range comprises 31 upper anterior moulds and 13 lower anterior moulds and the uppers are grouped into ovoid, tapering, square and rectangular.

The posterior teeth are available in three types: Cuspiform have anatomical occlusal surfaces with cusp inclination of 23–28° and optimum degree of inter-cuspation; Synoform has abraded occlusal surfaces, low degree of inter-cuspation and narrower posteriors; Lingoform are suitable for lingualised occlusion – the mandibular teeth have a buccal cusp inclination of 20° and 15° in the lingual area.

Physiodens: acrylic teeth

These are Vita's multilayered teeth that have opalescence and luminescence and are available in all 3D-Master and Classical shades as well as bleaching shades. The range consists of 20 upper anterior moulds, again grouped into ovoid, square, rectangular and tapering, combined with 8 lower anterior moulds and 6 posterior moulds or the Lingoform posteriors described above.

The Vita teeth can all be modified or characterised using the LC composite range.

Ivoclar Vivadent

SR Vivodent (acrylic)

This is an entry-level range with 25 upper anterior moulds and 10 lower moulds in 20 Chromoscope shades. The anterior teeth are combined with 5 upper and lower moulds in the SR Orthotype range.

SR Vivodent PE (acrylic)

This range consists of 24 upper and 8 lower anterior moulds in 20 Chromoscope shades. The teeth have improved aesthetics with a 'pearly appearance' and darker necks (Figure 216a). The material also gives rise to increased hardness and colour stability.

The teeth combine with either SR Orthosit PE posterior teeth (Figure 216b) or SR Othotype PE that have functional abrasion areas. All are produced using highly cross-linked Isosit dental material and are available in 20 shades and posterior moulds: 5-N, 2-K, 2-T.

SR Vivodent DCL (double cross-linked)

These anterior teeth are available in A1–D4, Chromoscope and additional bleaching shades in 24 upper anterior moulds and 8 lower anterior moulds (Figure 216c). The material demonstrates improved wear resistance and colour stability.

The anterior moulds combine with one of four types of posterior tooth mould, either SR Postaris DCL suggested for partial dentures and complete dentures, SR Orthotyp DCL (Figure 216d) for complete dentures, SR Ortholingual DCL (Figure 216e) for lingualised occlusion, or SR Orthoplane DCL (Figure 216f) for gerodontics. These latter teeth have reduced cusp height and are designed to allow horizontal movement of the mandible without interference.

SR Phonares NHC (nano hybrid composite)

Ivoclar's composite range of teeth include 18 upper anterior moulds grouped first into soft or bold and then each group subdivided into youthful, universal and mature.

The youthful moulds have no wear and an unabraided incisal edge, whereas the universal moulds have a slightly abraded incisal edge and reduced labial curvature. Finally, the mature group demonstrates heavy abrasion and flat labial surfaces.

The teeth feature wide tooth necks to help cover metal substructures and have concave distal margins and concave mesial margins to assist in setting the teeth and avoiding dark areas interproximally.

These teeth are produced from a UDMA (urethane dimethacrylate) matrix containing inorganically filled UDMA polymer, PMMA silanised SiO_2 nanoparticle and high-density silanised SiO_2, resulting in a material that demonstrates excellent wear and optical properties.

The teeth combine with either the SR Phonares Type NHC for conventional set-up with contacts between the upper palatal cusp and the lower buccal cusp or the SR Phonares Lingual NHC for lingualised occlusion teeth with contacts between the upper palatal cusps only.

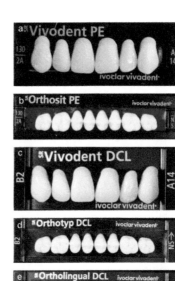
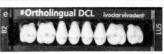
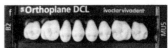

Figure 216

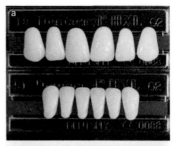

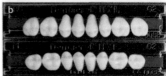

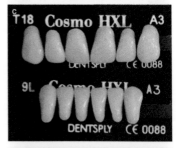

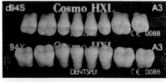

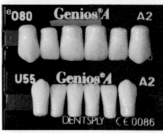

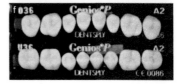

Figure 217

Dentacryl HXL (highly cross-linked)

These are the entry-level teeth in the Dentsply range with 15 upper and 5 lower anterior moulds (Figure 217a). Three types of posterior teeth are available: traditional, autoset, and special, the latter having reduced cusp angles (Figure 217b).

Cosmo HXL (highly cross-linked)

This tooth range has improved aesthetics over the Dentacryl range and splits the 20 upper anterior moulds into three groups: tapering, round and square, all of which are available in V-shades A1–D4, excluding C1 and B1 (Figure 217c). Seven lower anterior moulds are available to complement the various sizes of upper anteriors. The posterior teeth are available in five sizes and have a reduced cusp angle of 20° for easier setting (Figure 217d).

Genios

This range of teeth is produced in Dentsply's INPEN material (interpenetrated polymer network), resulting in better abrasion resistance and colour stability. The anterior teeth are produced in five layers, giving improved aesthetics and opalescence. They are designed to have reduced interdental space to reduce dark areas between teeth and to support the gingival acrylic and cover bars, attachments or clasps.

The range consists of nine upper anterior moulds and six lower anterior moulds available in V-shades A1–D4 (Figure 217e). The posterior teeth are available in five sizes, four of which are also available with a reduced ridge lap for limited space cases (Figure 217f).

Myerson

Three examples of Myerson teeth are shown in Figure 218. Each range is available in Vita Classic equivalent shades.

Myerson DB (dura-blend) plus

These resin anterior teeth are available in ovoid, tapered, square and rectangular mould forms with sizes ranging from approximately 40 mm up to 51 mm (distal–distal of the canine) (Figure 218a). The posterior teeth are composite and are available in 0°, 10°, 20° and 30° cusp angle versions. The 30° teeth are also available with reduced ridge lap for cases where vertical dimension is limited.

Myerson special

These teeth have greater characterisation, including darker necks to the teeth, a darker canine, enamel striation, translucent incisal areas, strong surface relief, decalcification areas, proximal stains and composite fillings (Figure 218b).

The anterior teeth are available in aesthetic, youthful and prime moulds. The aesthetic and youthful moulds are have tapered and square teeth whereas the prime are ovoid (Figure 218c).

In addition each are described by the manufacturer as follows.

- Aesthetic moulds: slender and subtle labial carving.
- Youthful moulds: shorter ridge lap, vigorous sculpting, and longer lingual line. Fewer striations.
- Prime moulds: for older patients, shorter, less sloping ridge lap, more pronounced age characteristics and curvature.

The posterior moulds, the Duratomic range, have a 30° cusp angle with simulated abrasion. They are available in four sizes – 28, 30, 32 and 34 mm (upper mesial of premolar to distal of second molar) – as shown in Figure 218d.

Myerson also offer a lingualised occlusion range – the Myerson Lingualised Intergration or mli range. These are available as MC or CC, the latter having reduced ridge lap (Figure 218e).

Myerson GanyMed

These are available in the same range as the specials, but are more heavily characterised and produced from a reinforced material (Figure 218f).

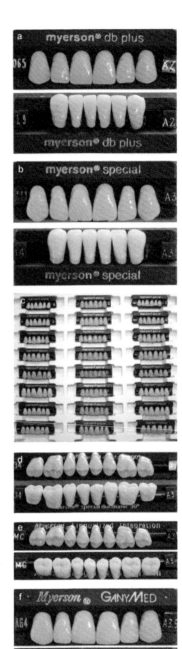

Figure 218

A price comparison between the denture teeth described in this section is shown in Table 2. The prices shown were correct at the time of publication but are obviously subject to constant change. Our reason for including this was to give the reader an idea of the comparative costs of the various teeth shown.

Table 2 Price comparison of a range of popular denture teeth from various manufacturers. The prices shown are in pounds Sterling and per set of denture teeth

	Upper anterior	Lower anterior	Upper posterior	Lower posterior	Total
Candulor					
Physioset TCR	15.66	15.66	12.99	12.99	57.30
Physiostar NFC	24.83	24.83	16.38	16.38	82.42
Physioset CT	21.39	21.39	12.80	12.80	68.38
Myerson					
db plus	6.15	6.15	6.15	6.15	24.60
Special	13.90	13.90	13.90	13.90	55.60
Gynamed	14.10	14.10	14.10	14.10	56.40
Schottlander					
Delphic V	2.68	2.68	2.00	2.00	9.36
Delphic	4.06	4.06	3.06	3.06	14.24
Natura	8.45	8.45	7.45	7.45	31.80
Enigma	15.95	15.95	13.50	13.50	58.90
Vita					
MFT	8.95	8.95	8.95	8.95	35.80
Physiodens	18.36	18.36	16.76	16.76	70.24
Vitapan	15.56	15.56	16.76	16.76	64.64
Ivoclar Vivodent					
Ivostar	5.08	5.08	5.08	5.08	20.32
SR Vivodent	7.95	7.95	7.95	7.95	31.80
SR Vivodent DCL	17.04	17.04	15.08	15.08	64.24
SR Vivodent PE	17.04	17.04	15.08	15.08	64.24
wDentsply					
Dentacryl	3.36	3.36	3.36	3.36	13.44
Cosmo HXL	4.95	4.95	4.95	4.95	19.80

Digital photography

Digital photography is hugely helpful in storing and communicating patient information. Existing dentures, patient face shape and profile, as well as before and after shots are invaluable in achieving satisfactory dentures.

For prosthetic work most modern digital cameras are capable of achieving a satisfactory portrait and profile picture.

To get the best from the camera:

- position your subject in a well-lit but not directly sunlit area;
- white balance the camera where available;
- select the portrait mode;
- if possible, mount the camera on a tripod with the flash off and take the shot using the self-timer. If no tripod is available, use flash ensuring that the white balance is set to 'flash'.

For close up shots, using a ring flash as shown in Figure 219a can produce well-balanced results that produce accurate colour and detail. Using the top flash on the camera may produce results with slightly burnt out colour and a loss of detail, as shown in Figure 219b.

Lighting the subject with natural light can produce results that are unbalanced because of the uneven fall of light onto the subject. This may not produce reliable colour or detail, as shown in Figure 220.

Old photographs

Old photographs showing the patient when they had their own teeth and are smiling are very valuable as a guide. The characteristics that they had in their natural teeth can be replicated in the denture teeth, with the patient's agreement (Figure 221a,b). The teeth can then be aged to match the patient's current age if a significant time difference exists between the age of the photograph and the patient's current age.

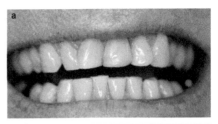
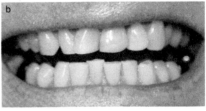

Figure 219

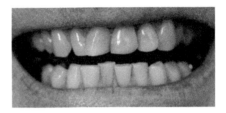

Figure 220

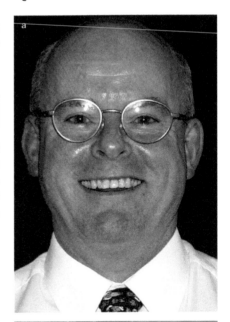
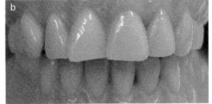

Figure 221

Chapter 7 | POSITIONING THE DENTURE TEETH

Creating a denture that is aesthetic, retentive and stable during function is challenging, however there are anatomical landmarks that can help in establishing the optimal position of the teeth.

The denture teeth should be positioned to create:

- an aesthetic appearance by siting the anterior teeth in a natural position relative to the alveolar, incisal papillae and lips (Figure 222);

- a stable denture by positioning the teeth over the central position of the alveolar ridges (Figure 223);

- stability during chewing by centring the primary chewing teeth over the most favourable part of the ridge (an analogy is seen with the position of a saddle on a horse's back as shown in Figure 224a. Marking the stable position on the patient's alveolar ridges, as shown in Figure 224b, will ensure that the large molar tooth is sited over this spot, as shown in Figure 224c, ensuring denture stability);

- stability of the lower denture by creating harmonious, non-antagonistic contacts between the mandibular and maxillary teeth during lateral and protrusive excursions (Figure 225a,b); and

- retention by ensuring that the denture teeth are held within the neutral zone or potential denture space, an area that exists between the forces exerted by the muscles of the cheeks, lips and tongue (Figure 226a,b).

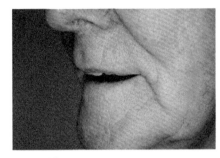

Figure 222

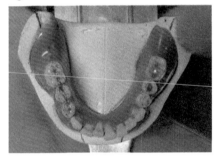

Figure 223

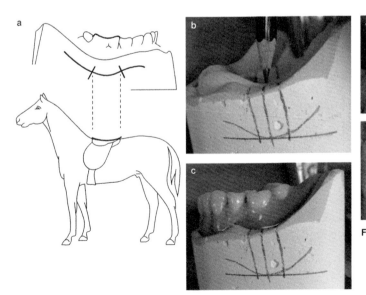
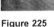

Figure 224

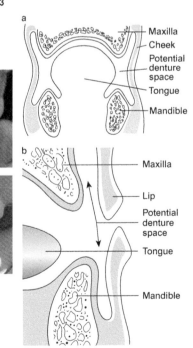

Figure 225

Figure 226

Techniques in Complete Denture Technology, First Edition. Tony Johnson, Duncan J. Wood.
© 2012 Tony Johnson and Duncan J. Wood. Published 2012 by Blackwell Publishing Ltd.

The shape, size and position of the anterior teeth provide the primary aesthetics of the denture. There are two occlusal schemes that may be used when designing the posterior tooth contact: balanced 'natural' or 'lingualised' occlusion. Each scheme uses the anatomical landmarks described above and below to determine the position of the teeth.

Anatomical landmarks and aids used to position denture teeth

Upper borders

- Midline: Reference plane to achieve anterior symmetry.
- Rugae: May be used to locate the canine.
- Tuberosity: Defines maximum posterior border of the occlusal table.
- Labial sulcus: Use to assess the vertical dimension.
- Hamular notch: Distal to the tuberosity, defines the maximum posterior border of the denture.
- Vibrating line: Position of post dam, the maximum distal border of the denture (foveae palatini).
- Alveolar ridge: Use to assess the bucco-palatal position of the teeth.

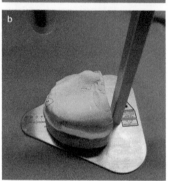

Figure 227

Lower borders

- Retromolar pad: Distal border of the lower denture. A point two-thirds the way up the retromolar pads may be used to approximate the occlusal plane.
- Labial sulcus: Use to assess vertical dimension.
- Alveolar ridge: Use to assess bucco-lingual position of lower teeth.
- Buccal shelf: Provides support for denture and angulation of occlusal surfaces of the posterior teeth.
- External oblique and mylohyoid ridges: Bony structures and muscle attachment sites that should not be included in denture-bearing area.

Incisal papillae

The incisal papilla is a key landmark in the design of the denture because it does not change position as the alveolar resorbs. The incisal papillae highlights the anatomical midline of the alveolar, regardless of the midline of the patient's face, as shown in Figure 227. The labial surface of the maxillary anterior teeth is approximately 8 mm anterior to the centre of the incisal papillae. This measurement can be used as a guide for placing the teeth (Figure 228a–c).

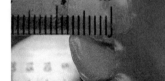

Figure 228

The position of the canines may also be related to the incisal papillae. The incisal tips should be in line with the centre of the incisal papillae as shown in Figure 229. Similarly, the labial surfaces of the canines are approximately 10 mm from the edge of the first rugae fold as an average position (Figure 230).

The position of the incisal papilla may be marked onto the occlusal registration rim using a laser and be used as an aid when positioning the anterior teeth (Figure 231a,b).

A simple device called an Alma gauge may also be used to accurately determine the labial contour of a registration rim, as shown in Figure 232. Here, the registration rim is placed on the device and the distance from the incisal papillae to the labial surface of the registration rim measured.

This device allows the patient's existing denture to be measured and the dimensions 'transferred' to a registration rim or trial denture (Figure 233). This quick procedure saves chairside time when adjusting registration rims and copies the position of well-placed teeth from existing dentures.

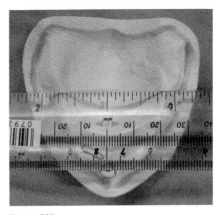

Figure 229

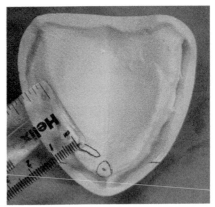

Figure 230

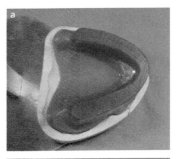

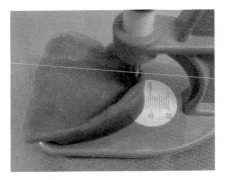

Figure 232

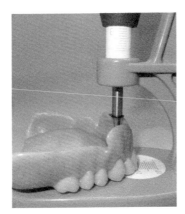

Figure 233

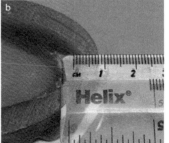

Figure 231

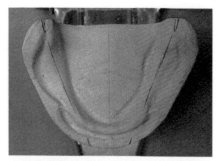

Figure 234

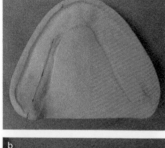

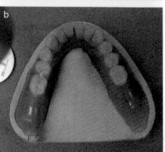

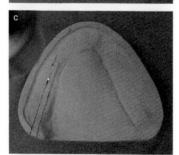

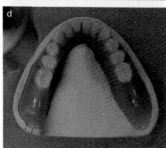

Figure 235

Alveolar ridge

Straight lines are often used between the retromolar pad and the first premolar to represent the centre of the alveolar ridge (Figure 234). Using the centre of the ridge may result in restricted tongue space if severe resorption of the ridges has taken place and the ridges have resorbed lingually, as shown in Figure 235a–d. This can lead to false tooth positioning and an unstable denture, which may be dislodged by the action of the tongue.

A better method is to first use a pencil or static laser to mark the centre of the denture-bearing area. In some cases this may be the crest of the alveolar ridge, but not always (see Figure 238a–c). This indicates the optimum position to be used as the bucco-lingual determinant of the teeth in both upper and lower arches (Figure 236).

When positioning the teeth, the use of a static laser or similar device as shown in Figure 237a,b is an excellent way to ensure the teeth are correctly centred over the most stable part of the denture-bearing area.

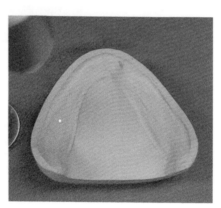

Figure 236

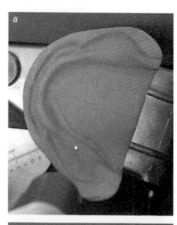

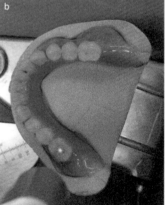

Figure 237

Correctly positioning posterior teeth is also significant in preventing fracture of the denture. When upper or lower posterior teeth are placed too far buccally the denture becomes susceptible to fracture because the occlusal forces are transmitted down the buccal aspects of the ridges rather than onto the crests of the ridges. This causes stress concentration at the midline of the denture. Figure 238a,b shows a laser used to identify the centre of the ridge (Figure 238a) and when the wax try-in denture is placed onto the model it can be seen that the denture teeth have been positioned too far buccally.

Saddle

To achieve stability, the occlusal force should be transmitted at 90° to the alveolar and the primary masticatory teeth should be located in the deepest part of the alveolar. (This is particularly important for the mandibular denture.)

As shown in Figure 239, the deepest part of the alveolar on the ridge is marked using a pencil and transcribed to the side of the model for use when positioning the lower molar.

A profile compass (Figure 240) may also be used to trace the contour of the ridge onto the side of the model to help prevent teeth being sited over sloping parts of ridges. The compass should be kept at right-angles to the alveolar when making this tracing.

Lines to indicate the posterior and anterior extent of the most stable part of the ridge (the part you would put the horse's saddle onto) are then drawn as shown in Figure 241. A combination of ridge profile and lowest point of the alveolar provide a guide for large molar placement. No occluding posterior teeth should be placed distal to the most posterior line as they would be over the sloping part of the ridge, which would cause instability during mastication. The primary masticatory tooth (the first molar) should be placed between the two lines as shown in Figure 242a,b. Never place molar teeth over the distal, sloping, parts of ridges. If this means leaving the last molar off the denture so be it. A more stable, better functioning denture will result!

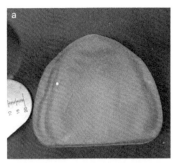

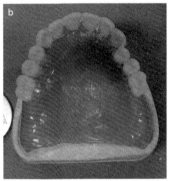

Figure 238

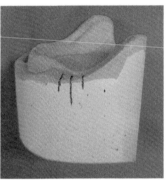

Figure 239

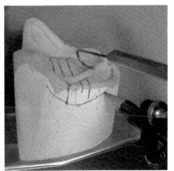

Figure 240

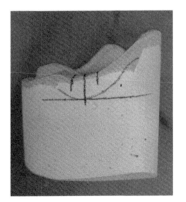

Figure 241

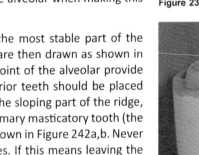

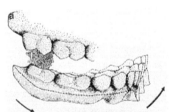

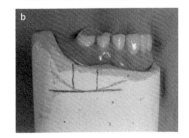

Figure 242

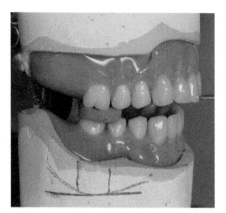

Figure 243

This becomes significant in providing stability for the denture once food is between the teeth. When a bolus of food is being chewed, balanced occlusion is lost and the teeth must be designed such that they are unilaterally stable. As shown in Figure 243, correctly positioned molar teeth will allow masticatory pressure, exerted during eating, to be transferred through the dentures and help to stabilise the denture rather than dislodge it as would be the case if the molar teeth were over sloping ridges.

Studies show that chewing takes place for approximately 15 minutes per day. It is during this function that we require the unilateral stability. We can rely on retention when dentures are new, but as they lose their good adaptation, due to resorption of tissue and bone, so retention is reduced and stability becomes important.

Retaining the registration information

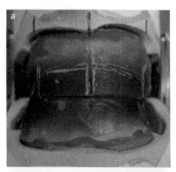

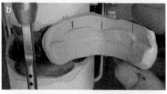

When positioning teeth in the registration rim, the information recorded onto the rim is lost. The centre line and canine lines are easily transferred to the models, but the smile lines and sagittal contour of the incisors are less easy to store. As shown in Figure 244a–c, the details recorded on the labial surface of maxillary registration rims, centre line, smile line and labial contour can be recorded using impression putty and used to verify correct placement of the teeth.

Design of the occlusion

There are two forms of posterior tooth relationship for complete dentures: the natural/anatomical balanced occlusion and the lingualised occlusion. Although these are similar, the lingualised occlusion has a much smaller number of contacts between the upper and lower teeth. This allows more control of the pressure directed through the dentures onto the underlying supporting tissues.

The natural/anatomical occlusion

Figure 244

The upper teeth are placed in their natural position, slightly buccal to the crest of the ridge (Figure 245). Typically, these teeth are placed starting from the first premolar through to the second molar, creating compensating curves relative to the occlusal plane. As shown in Figure 246, the compensating curve, a combination of the curves of Spee and Monson or Wilson, can be built into the posterior arrangement of the denture teeth.

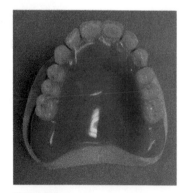

Figure 245

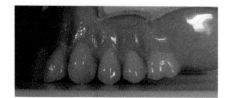

Figure 246

Occlusal contacts are established between the buccal cusps of the lower teeth and the central fossae of the upper, and the palatal cusps of the upper teeth and the central fossae of the lower as illustrated by Figure 247a–d. The teeth also overlap each other in a natural manner; the lower first premolar occluding with the upper canine and first premolar, the lower second premolar occluding with the upper first and second premolars, and the lower molar occluding with the upper second premolar and first molar.

In natural occlusion dentures the teeth overlap each other and replicate nature as shown in Figure 248. Note that the second molar should only be placed if there is room to do so without encroaching onto the sloping part of the lower ridge. In this case it would occlude with the upper first and second molars.

In lateral excursions, contact of the working side cusps is maintained. Therefore the lower buccal cusp tip translates down the palatal facing slope of the upper buccal cusp. The upper palatal cusp remains in contact with the buccal facing slope of the lower lingual cusp as shown in Figure 249a,b. Simultaneously on the balancing side, the upper palatal cusps slides up the lingual facing slope of the lower buccal cusps (Figure 250).

In protrusive excursions, as shown in Figure 251, anterior and posterior contacts are maintained during protrusive excursions to prevent the denture from tipping.

When establishing an occlusal scheme in this way, there are many contacts to consider, which must all be harmonised with the movements of the mandible. The articulator should be programmed to best replicate the mandibular movements in order that the teeth may be engineered to match the patient's condylar pathway.

There is little room for error and the teeth are generally designed to have a precise 'centric' position. This means that the inter-cuspal position (ICP) contacts established to coincide with centric relation are single points to which the patient must close.

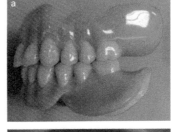
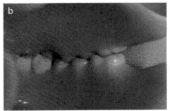
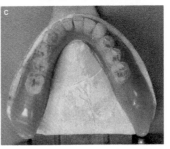
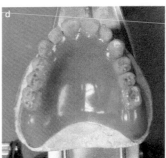

Figure 247

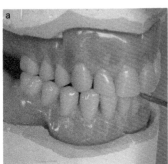

Figure 249

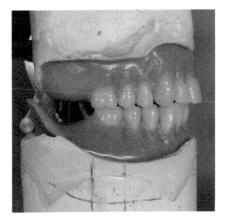

Figure 248

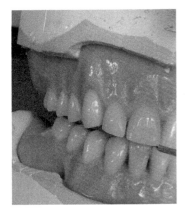

Figure 250

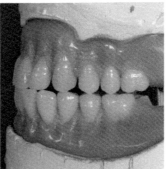

Figure 251

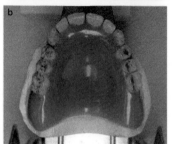
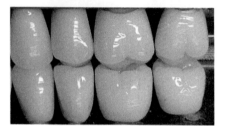

Figure 252

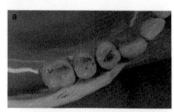

Figure 253

Lingualised occlusion

The lingualised occlusion is designed to direct the occlusal forces over the centre of the alveolar using one contact per tooth. This simplifies the tooth contacts by eliminating the buccal cusp contact. The resulting occlusal contacts are lingually placed in comparison to the natural occlusion.

Lingualised occlusion teeth have far fewer occlusal contacts then their natural occlusion counterparts. Figure 252a,b shows lingualised occlusion teeth on the patient's left.

In lingualised occlusion dentures the teeth are designed with large maxillary palatal cusps that occlude with enlarged opposing fossae (Figure 253). During excursions, the single occlusal contacts are harmonised with the movement of the condyle in each direction, creating a pestle and mortar style of occlusion (Figure 254a,b).

The centric contacts are wider and longer than found in natural teeth, allowing a degree of tolerance when the denture wearer occludes the teeth, as shown in Figure 255.

Importantly, the single contact per tooth is centred directly over the alveolar ridge to create stability. With the lower teeth dictating the lingual–buccal position, the upper teeth, having more tolerance due to the broader upper ridge, are generally placed buccal to the upper ridge (Figure 256).

Occlusal contact occurs between the palatal cusps of the upper teeth and the central fossae of the lower teeth (see Figure 253). The first premolars have this situation reversed (Figure 257a,b).

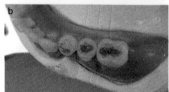

Figure 254

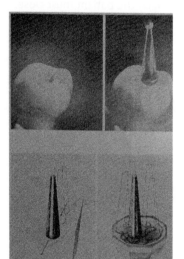

Figure 255

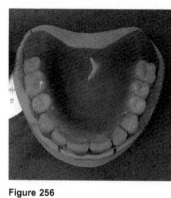

Figure 256

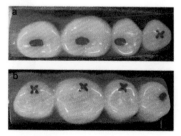

Figure 257

No overlapping of the teeth is introduced, the upper tooth only occludes with its lower counterpart (see Figure 253). With no contact between the buccal cusps of the teeth, the occlusal contacts are lingually placed in comparison to the natural occlusion. This means that the forces are directed over the lower ridge, resulting in the most favourable situation for mechanical stability. This form of occlusion is indicated where the alveolar ridge is less pronounced and stability of the denture is paramount.

It should be remembered that although centric relation and the movements of the mandible may be recorded precisely, these positions and movements are subject to change throughout the day or over time. The difference in centric relation over a 24-hour period has been demonstrated, and change over time may result from a number of causes, including relaxing of the muscles if they have been working from a poor position previously, remodelling of the condylar head, or reduction of inflammation.

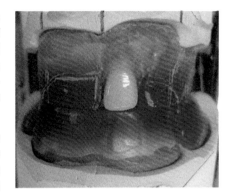

Figure 258

Whatever the reason, it may be considered that the best long-term treatment is to provide an occlusal scheme that will allow the patient to adjust and move freely while still maintaining a stable denture.

With the 'one cusp into one fossa' arrangement of the teeth with this method, it is possible to create a 'long and wide centric' situation to allow patients a freedom in centric. Similarly those who have problems achieving the same occlusal position habitually will be able to maintain balanced occlusion. During the final grinding-in of the teeth, a balanced occlusion can be achieved even if the patient makes a protrusive or retrusive shift of 2–3 mm.

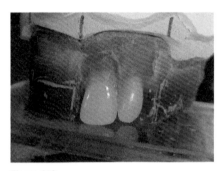

Figure 259

Setting teeth in natural occlusion

When setting the teeth in natural occlusion, first an upper central incisor is placed to one side of the centre line, replacing the labial contour of the upper wax block, and just touching the occlusal plane (Figure 258). Then the lower rim or a glass slab placed against the upper block is used to indicate the occlusal plane.

The lateral incisor should be positioned with the incisal edge 0–2 mm off the occlusal plane. (This will vary according to the age of the patient; older patients would not normally be expected to have a 'youthful' step, as shown in Figure 259, between their centrals and laterals, due to wear of the centrals and canines.)

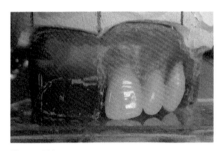

Figure 260

The centrals and laterals should have their incisal edges placed more anteriorly than their necks to support the lips in a slightly prominent and natural position. The canines should be positioned to show their mesial aspects when viewed from the front, and the incisal edge should just touch the occlusal plane (Figure 260).

The distal aspect should be pointing down the wax blocks to link into the posterior teeth and create a natural looking buccal corridor. The neck of the canine should be prominent and more anteriorly placed than the incisal edge to emphasise the canine eminence and to support the lips (Figure 261). By setting up one entire side of the anterior teeth first, rather than two centrals followed by two laterals and finally two canines, the labial contour of the block can be maintained until one side is correctly positioned.

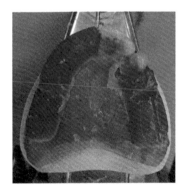

Figure 261

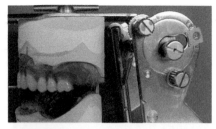

Figure 262

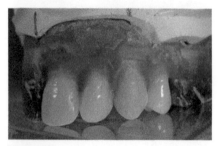

Figure 263

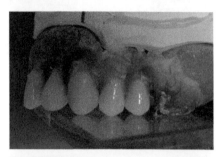

Figure 264

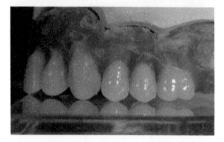

Figure 265

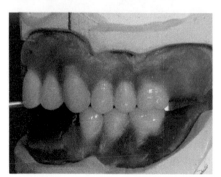

Figure 266

Class I

The upper posterior teeth are set over or slightly buccal to the ridge, such that their occlusal surfaces lie slightly buccal to the lower ridge (see Figure 245). The teeth are positioned to create a compensating curve (see Figure 246). The steepness of the curve depends on the condylar angle, the cusp angle of the teeth and incisal guidance table angle. The steeper the angle, the steeper the compensating curve needs to be. The curve of Spee, antero-posterior curve of the posterior teeth, should match the condylar angle to maintain contact between the teeth in protrusive excursions as shown in Figure 262.

The upper first premolar is positioned with palatal and buccal cusps contacting the occlusal plane. The long axis of the tooth is vertical when observed from the buccal aspect (Figure 263). The second premolar is positioned, again with a vertical long axis when viewed buccally, but with the buccal cusp lifted slightly off the occlusal plane by 0.5–1 mm. Only the palatal cusp touches the occlusal plane (Figure 264).

The first molar tooth is positioned again with the mesiopalatal cusp contacting the occlusal surface and the remaining cusps lifted to continue the compensating curve started by the second premolar. As shown in Figure 265 the mesio-palatal cusp is the nearest to the occlusal plane and the disto-buccal cusp the furthest away.

The lower molar tooth is positioned to occlude with the upper such that the mesio-palatal cusp of the upper tooth occludes with the central fossae of the lower tooth. The lower second premolar is placed to occlude with the upper second and first premolars. Finally, the first premolars are placed to occlude with the upper first premolar and the distal aspect of the canine (Figure 266).

The second molar teeth should only be placed if there is room to do so without placing them over the sloping parts of the ridges, which would cause denture instability. In Figure 267, placing the last molar tooth would mean it was over a sloping part of the mandibular ridge so it has been omitted.

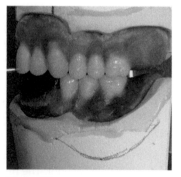

Figure 267

Lower anterior teeth

Lower anterior teeth should be positioned to create an arbitrary 1–2 mm overjet and overbite where possible. Always remember to ensure that the forces generated when incising food are directed down through the anterior teeth onto the alveolar ridges, which effectively pushes the dentures against the ridges for maximum support (Figure 268a,b).

Class II

This is a posterior relationship of the mandible to the maxilla and with natural teeth the mesio-buccal cusp of the first upper permanent molar occludes mesial to the mesio-buccal groove of the lower first permanent molar. In complete dentures a normal relationship is maintained between the upper and lower posterior teeth. However, because the lower arch is narrower than the upper arch, because of the posterior relationship of the mandible to the maxilla, a normal relationship between the upper and lower teeth cannot usually be achieved if the teeth are to be placed over the most stable parts of the upper and lower ridges. To achieve a reasonable occlusal relationship, while maintaining the teeth in the most stable position over the ridges, the central fossae of the lower posterior teeth must be extended buccally by grinding, to allow contact between the upper palatal cusps and the lower buccal fossae (Figure 269). This usually means there is no contacts between the upper buccal cusps and the lower palatal cusps with their antagonists, which would be the case in a class I relationship. It also means that a much larger buccal overjet is seen than normal, as shown in Figure 270.

Lower anterior teeth

Class II set-ups usually exhibit reduced space for the mandibular incisors. It is better to place five anterior teeth of the correct size to match the maxillary teeth (Figure 271a) than to select too small a set of mandibular teeth. Alternatively, it is sometimes better aesthetically to leave off the first premolars and replace them with mandibular canines, which can be placed to articulate better with the maxillary first premolar. The aesthetics are also improved even if seven mandibular anterior teeth are placed (Figure 271b,c). One extra tooth or one less tooth will not usually be noticed by anyone looking at the patient.

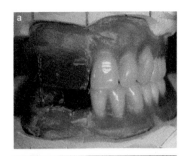
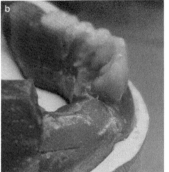

Figure 268

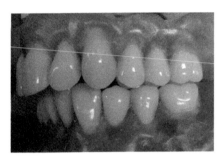

Figure 269

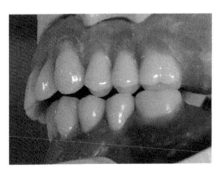

Figure 270

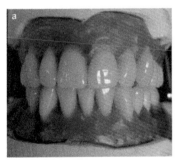
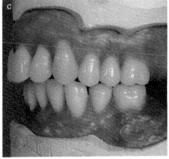
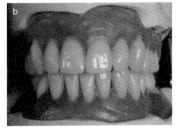

Figure 271

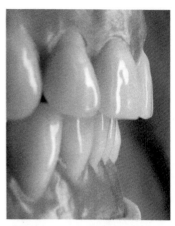

Figure 272

The overjet and overbite are inevitably larger than the usual 2 mm recommendation (Figure 272). However, it is important that the lower teeth remain in the neutral zone and that occlusal forces are directed down the long axis of the teeth onto the lower ridges, maintaining stability of the denture. It is still possible to achieve this by proclining the teeth forwards slightly to enable an edge-to-edge relationship of the incisor teeth during biting. In these class II cases it is sometimes tempting to position the lower teeth too far forwards to try to allow better contact between the anterior teeth during protrusive/biting excursions. This can lead to instability when incising food because the biting forces are not directed back onto the ridges. Labially placed teeth may also interfere with the movement of the lower lip, particularly as it moves when pronouncing 'E' sounds.

Class III

This is an anterior relationship of the mandible to the maxilla. In natural teeth the mesio-buccal cusp of the upper first permanent molar occludes distal to the mesio-buccal groove of the lower first permanent molar. In class III complete denture cases, the lower arch is usually wider than the upper arch because of the anterior relationship of the mandible to the maxilla. In complete denture class III cases a normal relationship between the posterior teeth is maintained (Figure 273).

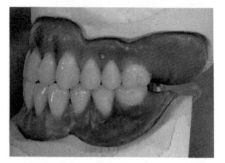

Figure 273

However, a crossbite situation frequently occurs in this classification, and this can either be unilateral or bilateral. When crossbites occur, the buccal cusps of the upper teeth are used to occlude with the central fossae of the lower teeth (Figure 274). This is perfectly normal and crossbites should be set up in situations where providing a normal relationship would mean placing the teeth off the centre of the ridges, which would cause instability during function. Attempts should not be made to turn these cases into class I relationships.

In crossbite cases the necks of the upper posterior teeth should be extended buccally and the waxwork slightly overbuilt to support the cheeks and prevent them from falling into the buccal surfaces of the lower teeth and being bitten during function (Figure 275).

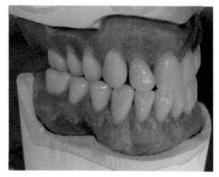

Figure 274

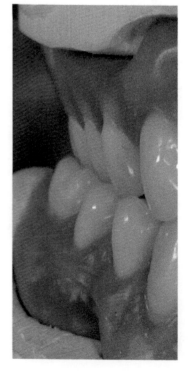

Figure 275

Lower anterior teeth

This situation is the direct opposite of that seen for the class II cases. An edge-to-edge contact is seen between the upper and lower anterior teeth. This usually also sees a situation where the space left for the lower anterior teeth is greater than the width of the teeth chosen to match the upper anterior teeth. As with the class II anterior teeth, keeping the correct size ratio between upper and lower anterior teeth, and having extra numbers of teeth, rather than wider ones, maintains better aesthetics. It is better to have seven proportionally matching teeth than to place six larger teeth that are the wrong relationship to the maxillary anteriors (Figure 276). However, in some severe cases this is not possible while still allowing the forces down the long axis of the teeth during eating to be directed onto the lower ridges. Many technicians ignore this and provide dentures that tip when the patient bites through food. In these severe cases it is better to copy what would have been the natural situation and place the lower anterior teeth slightly anterior to the upper teeth to allow pressure directed down through the lower anterior teeth to be directed onto the lower ridge during the incising of food (Figure 277).

Setting teeth in lingualised occlusion

The upper anterior teeth are positioned as previously described for natural occlusion (see Figures 258–261). When using lingualised occlusion, the lower posterior teeth are usually positioned first.

Class I

The contour of the lower ridge is drawn along the side of the model using an adapted compass (Figure 278). The occlusal plane of the lower posterior teeth should conform to the curve of the lower ridge with the first molar tooth positioned to be over the lowest point of the ridge (Figure 279). This can sometimes lead to a shortened occlusal table as shown in Figure 280.

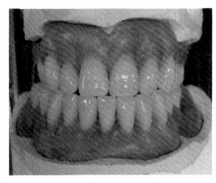

Figure 276

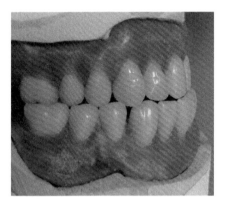

Figure 277

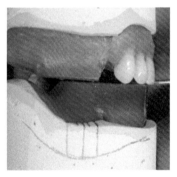

Figure 278

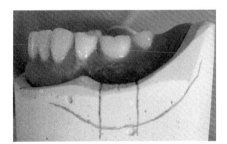

Figure 280

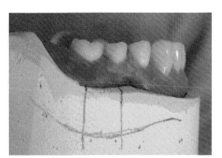

Figure 279

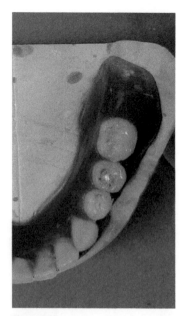

Figure 281

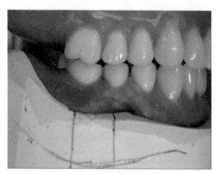

Figure 282

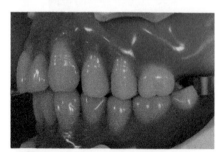

Figure 283

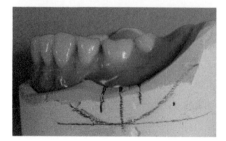

Figure 284

The height of the occlusal plane may need to be adjusted carefully to ensure that the upper posterior teeth do not appear to be hanging down below the upper anterior teeth when the patient opens their mouth or smiles. Ensure that the central fossae of the lower posterior teeth are directly over the centre of the lower ridge with a static laser (Figure 281).

The upper posterior teeth can then be positioned. The teeth are positioned so that the large palatal cusps of the second premolar and first molar occlude with the large central fossae of their lower counterparts. This situation is reversed with the first premolars, where the large buccal cusp of the lower first premolar occludes with the central fossa of the upper first premolar. Figure 282 illustrates that no overlap of the posterior teeth is seen in lingualised occlusion set-ups.

The teeth should be positioned so that they are directing forces at right-angles to the ridge. This may mean that they deviate slightly from the occlusal plane and do not conform to the 'normal' compensating curve. The occlusal plane is used only to regulate the correct height of the posterior teeth (Figure 283).

Ideally the largest posterior tooth, the first molar, should be placed over the most stable part of the mandibular ridge (the best analogy for this is a saddle on a horses back) as shown in Figure 284.

As previously mentioned, this arrangement of the teeth can often lead to fewer posterior teeth being placed compared to the natural occlusion (Figure 285). There are a number of options that can be employed in these circumstances.

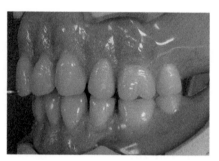

Figure 285

- To aid the stability of the denture during protrusive movements a reversed first premolar – a 'spare' premolar – can be placed behind the last lower molar. This tooth is not in occlusion during normal masticatory excursions but will occlude with the upper molar during protrusive excursions and when incising through food. This negates the effect of Christensen's phenomenon (a dis-occlusion of the posterior teeth in protrusive excursions) and provides balanced occlusion in this excursion (Figure 286).

- To increase the size of the occlusal table an upper first premolar can be substituted for the upper canine. The lower canine is then positioned to occlude with the central fossa of this tooth. By angling the premolar outwards a little more than usual for a canine it is possible to 'hide' the palatal cusp and make this tooth to all intents and purposes a 'canine' (Figure 287a,b). This usually has no detrimental effect of aesthetics.

- It is also possible to substitute the molars for premolars. This has the effect of increasing the occlusal table. Also. by reducing the bucco-lingual width of the teeth, it makes then more efficient at cutting through the food bolus. They therefore exert less pressure on the underlying tissue and bone (Figure 288).

The lower anterior teeth are positioned according to the lower ridge and upper anterior teeth. Function should normally be given preference over aesthetics. Therefore accommodation may need to be made when placing the lower anterior teeth to maintain denture stability.

Although the overjet and overbite should not be exaggerated, it is important that the lower teeth remain in the neutral zone and are not positioned to create an arbitrary 1–2 mm overjet and overbite.

It should be noted that dentures made using this technique may not be symmetrical about the midline. This is of little consequence and is a result of following the anatomical structures of the mouth.

Class II

Class II relationships inevitably mean that when positioning the premolar teeth the lower premolars are positioned more lingually than would be the case for class I or III cases. This usually means that the central fossa of the upper first premolar has to be enlarged palatally to allow the lower premolar to contact it while still being positioned over the crest of the lower ridge.

The remaining teeth may also need to be adjusted. The central fossa of the lower second premolar and molar teeth may need to be adjusted to be more buccally placed, to allow correct positioning of the teeth over the ridges and contact between the teeth. There is always more 'leeway' when placing the upper teeth because the upper ridge is wider than the lower.

The room for the lower anterior teeth in class II cases is usually reduced compared to class I and III cases. It is much better to place five anterior teeth of the correct size than to try to place six teeth that are too small.

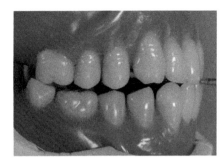

Figure 286

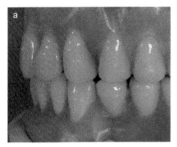

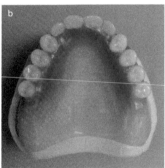

Figure 287

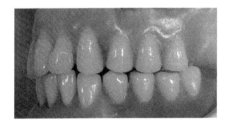

Figure 288

Class III

Class III jaw relationships are nearly the reverse of the class II situation. The lower jaw is usually wider than the upper jaw, which means that in a large number of cases either a unilateral or bilateral crossbite situation is encountered. In this situation the lower posterior teeth are positioned over the ridges as normal. The upper teeth are positioned over the ridges in such a way that the buccal cusps occlude with the central fossa of their lower counterparts. To prevent cheek biting during mastication, a common problem for class III patients, the upper posterior teeth are tilted outwards to make the necks of the teeth more prominent and buccally placed than the cusps. This has the effect of keeping the cheeks away from the occlusal surfaces and also allows better contact between the upper buccal cusp and the lower central fossa.

To improve the contact between the teeth, a central fossa may need to be 'created' on the lower first premolar for the upper first premolars buccal cusp to sit into (if finances allow it is sometimes better to substitute the first premolars for second premolars in these cases). All the upper buccal cups of the posterior teeth may need to be slightly rounded and the lower tooth ground to widen the fossa to accept the upper buccal cusps. If the palatal cusps prevent lateral movement, the tooth should be inclined to prevent the contact or the cusp reduced slightly by grinding.

In extreme cases, the upper canines can be replaced by premolars to ensure that there is adequate tooth contact and bring the occlusal table forward (see Figure 287a,b).

Limiting the occlusal table

The occlusal table is the area of functional tooth contact. Attempting to reproduce the natural occlusal table on prosthesis appears to make sense but often causes instability of the denture due to the unstable loading of the teeth posteriorly. A good analogy for this is when wearing skis and standing on a sloping surface, inevitably you start to move down the slope! When denture teeth that are placed over the sloping aspects of the posterior lower ridges are loaded with food bolus, the inevitable movement of the denture is forwards down the slope! Leaving teeth off this part of the denture leads to better denture stability (see Figure 242a,b).

As a general rule, the second molar teeth should not be incorporated into the denture unless they can be placed over a flat, stable, part of the lower ridge.

Dealing with limited space

Placing the posterior teeth in the most stable position often leads to a 'shortened dental arch' situation. Positioning the large first molar tooth first in the lower arch can lead to reduced room for the premolars and lower anterior teeth. This can frequently lead to a situation where only one premolar can be placed in front of the molar. This is not a problem as the major consideration when setting up the teeth, particularly the lower ones, should be the stability of the denture.

To try and increase the length of the occlusal table the upper canine can be exchanged for a second premolar. The lower canine can then be set to occlude with the central fossa of this tooth, thereby increasing the length of the functional occlusal table as shown in Figure 287a,b.

A simple alternative is to omit a premolar tooth and leave a small gap distal to an intact canine.

Providing stability in protrusive excursions

In situations where a large overjet is present, it may be necessary to provide additional teeth to ensure stability in the protrusive excursion. A premolar can be positioned behind the lower molar to ensure that a posterior contact is maintained during protrusion to the 'edge-to-edge' relationship of the anterior teeth (see Figure 286). This situation can be created in both class I and class II cases and is particularly useful for class II skeletal relationships where a large overjet is present. It is routinely useful where the patient's condylar angles have not been recorded and may be larger then 30°, leading to a 'Christensen's phenomenon' type situation being created in protrusive excursions.

Stability

In many cases lower denture stability is a problem, so to provide the optimal occlusal stability the posterior teeth can be set to be parallel to the contour of the lower ridge rather than at right-angles to the occlusal plane (see Figure 284). This ensures that the force exerted through the lower denture is always at right-angles to the ridge and helps to stabilise the denture rather than dislodge it.

Chapter 8 | GINGIVAL CONTOURING AND POLISHED SURFACES

Dentures replace teeth, resorbed bone and the surrounding soft tissue. The denture base that replaces the bone and tissues should be aesthetic, hygienic and contoured to harmonise with the muscles, Ideally, it should also be shaped such that retention and stability are helped.

Each denture must be designed individually by reading the signs on the model and by having knowledge of the muscles that surround the denture.

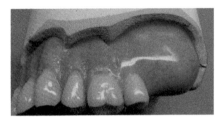

Figure 289

Sulcus

Filling the sulcus with the denture base provides the optimal seal around the denture, aiding retention. As shown in Figure 289, with fully functional impressions/models the denture base should be extended fully into the sulcus to achieve a good seal between the denture periphery and the tissues.

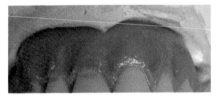

Figure 290

Care should be taken to ensure that the sulcus is not overbuilt, particularly in the upper anterior region where alveolar loss is less and excessive material conspicuous. As shown in Figure 290, the labial peripheries of dentures should not be over-contoured, as the sulcus in these areas does not resorb as much as other areas of the mouth. Thus the labial surfaces should be contoured to create 'lip shields' for the orbicularis oris muscle, which is the sphincter muscle around the mouth that may easily displace a lower denture. The denture should also be designed with the lower teeth over the alveolar ridge with the labial flange extending fully into the labial sulcus. A partial neutral zone denture technique could be helpful in shaping this important area of the denture base and may make it easier to position the mandibular teeth by providing an anatomical guide (Figure 291).

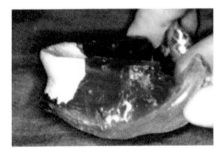

Figure 291

Denture base

Once the teeth are secured in position, all areas of the denture base, particularly those distal to the molars, which are regularly removed during the registration stage, should be replaced using wax. This non-occluding part of the denture will allow the tongue to brace the lower denture if properly contoured.

Techniques in Complete Denture Technology, First Edition. Tony Johnson, Duncan J. Wood.
© 2012 Tony Johnson and Duncan J. Wood. Published 2012 by Blackwell Publishing Ltd.

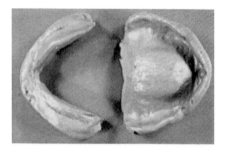

Figure 292

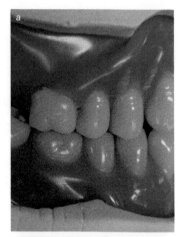

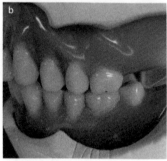

Figure 293

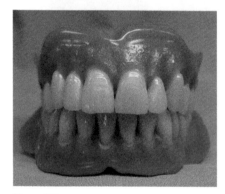

Figure 294

Buccal and lingual flange extension

The width of the buccal and lingual flanges on both upper and lower dentures should be constructed to fit fully into the sulci of the working models, which should have been produced from fully functional impressions, such as the mucocompressive impressions shown in Figure 292. Dentures made on models constructed from non-functional impressions will have flanges that do not conform to those of the patient and will at best be a 'guess' by the technician and clinician and in all probability fail clinically.

Care should be taken to ensure that the flange does not encroach onto the buccal or lingual frenulum. It is important to remember that the posterior buccal frenulum lies in a posterior direction when at rest. The denture base should be contoured to accept the frenulum in these positions, which should aid denture retention (Figure 293a,b).

Buccal and lingual flange contour (polished surface shape)

The contour of the buccal and lingual flanges, or the 'polished surfaces' of the denture, can have a major effect on denture stability (see Chapter 11 on neutral zone dentures). A good appreciation of the actions of the muscles of mastication is essential when contouring the polished surfaces of the dentures. Figures 294 shows labial contouring of the denture to harmonise with the muscles of mastication, for example, and Figure 295 shows fully contoured dentures, which take into account the muscles of mastication, allowing the muscles to act with the denture contours to help keep the denture in place.

Figure 296 shows the distribution and anticipated action of the muscles of mastication, starting from the node of the cheek muscles, which points out the necessity of shaping the base so that the muscles can grip it. The muscles shown in Figure 296 and their influence on the denture bases are as follows.

- The levator anguli oris and depressor anguli oris (c+d) pull in the direction of the cheek ligaments.

- The zygomatic muscle (e) pulls with parts of the buccinator (g) towards the zygomatic ridge.

- The risorius (f) also runs backwards with parts of the buccinator (g) towards the diagonal.

- The masseter muscle (m) overlaps the cheek eminence towards the back of the mouth.

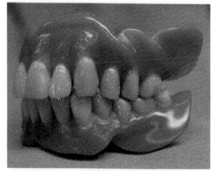

Figure 295

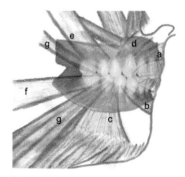

Figure 296

The lingual surfaces of the lower denture should be shaped to provide maximum room for the tongue in such a way as to allow the tongue to rest on the denture base and direct forces such that they help to retain it in contact with the underlying tissues and bone and not dislodge it (see Chapter 11 on neutral zone dentures).

Palate

The palate should generally be smooth and extend to the junction of the hard and soft palate. The shape of the anterior palate can have a significant effect on speech and this should be assessed and modified at the try-in stage by the clinician and technician. Artificial rugae may be provided relatively easily using a silicone impression of the patient's own rugae to aid in sculpting the wax (Figure 297). Smooth dentures are easier to clean, and some patients who have worn smooth palate dentures for a long time may find such features an irritant. However, they may be worth considering if difficulty is being experienced with phonetics. The undulating surfaces may allow a more natural contact with the tongue and aid word formation. The formed rugae should be smooth so they do not irritate the tongue, collect food debris or encourage plaque accumulation.

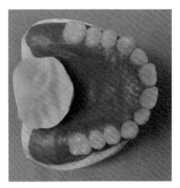

Figure 297

Gingival contour

Sculpting the wax around the teeth can affect aesthetics and hygiene. The gingival area should be sculptured to create an as aesthetic and natural situation as possible. Older patients, for example, would be expected to have receding gum levels, and although filling embrasures with pink acrylic would certainly allow the dentures to be cleaned readily, it would look false for an elderly patient. So a degree of compromise is needed to create a gingiva that reflects the tooth arrangement and the patient's age but still allows the denture to be relatively self-cleaning or easily cleaned by the patient. The denture wax-up in Figure 298 shows a typically youthful patient's gingival margin on the right hand side of the photograph, and a typical example of an older patient's gingival margin on the left. Note that in both cases the gingiva is symmetrical and smooth to allow ease of cleaning by the patient.

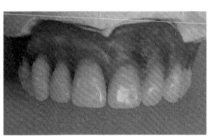

Figure 298

Chapter 9 | PROCESSING DENTURES

Processing a denture from the try-in to the finished acrylic denture is a technique-sensitive stage in the production of dental prosthesis. Polymethyl methacrylate (PMMA) has good aesthetic properties and is cheap and easy to process, but it is prone to contraction during processing. When considering the requirements of a denture base material, the list is extensive, and it is clear to see why there have been few alternative choices available.

Ideal properties

The ideal denture base material would have the following properties:

- natural appearance;
- reasonable strength, stiffness, hardness and toughness;
- dimensionally stability;
- absence of odour, taste or toxic products;
- resistance to absorbance of oral fluids;
- good retention to polymers, porcelain and metal;
- easy to repair;
- good shelf life;
- easy to manipulate;
- low density;
- accurate reproduction of surface detail;
- resistant to bacterial growth;
- good thermal conductivity;
- radio opaque;
- easy to clean;
- inexpensive to use;
- the ability to be stained/coloured to match individual patient gingiva.

Techniques in Complete Denture Technology, First Edition. Tony Johnson, Duncan J. Wood.
© 2012 Tony Johnson and Duncan J. Wood. Published 2012 by Blackwell Publishing Ltd.

Acrylic types

There are various types of acrylic available that can be used, most of which are either heat-cured or cold-cured.

Heat-cured acrylics

Powdered forms are beads or granules of polymethyl methacrylate:

- initiator – benzoyl peroxide,
- pigments,
- opacifiers – titanium or zinc oxides,
- plasticisers – dibutyl phthalate,
- synthetic fibres – nylon or acrylic.

Liquid forms are methyl methacrylate monomer:

- inhibitor – hydroquinone,
- cross-linking agent – ethylene glycol dimethacrylate.

The use of the polymer allows dough to be produced for processing, reduces shrinkage on polymerisation and minimises the exothermic reaction.

Cold-cured acrylics

The chemistry of these materials is the same as that for heat-cured materials, with the exception of the initiator, which is dimethyl-*p*-toluidine. Curing is less efficient, resulting in a lower molecular weight (lower density of cross-linking), compromising the mechanical properties and leaving residual monomer in the resin. Colour stability is also compromised.

High-impact heat-cured acrylics

These include a rubber-toughening agent such as a fine dispersion of butadiene styrene. These inclusions prevent crack propagation, resulting in a higher degree of resistance to fracture.

The impact strength of these materials can be almost tenfold more than that of conventional heat-cured acrylics. The adverse consequence is that they also lower the flexural modulus, and long-term fatigue failure due to excessive flexure can be a problem.

These materials are not widely used due to their greater cost.

Processing problems

Powder/liquid ratio

Too much polymer can result in inadequate softening of the powder by the monomer, resulting in a weak material. Too much monomer will result in excessive polymerisation shrinkage, loss of fit and increased potential for gaseous porosity.

Contraction porosity

This phenomenon is associated with polymerisation shrinkage. It occurs because the monomer contracts by 20% of its volume during curing. This is minimised by the use of a powder/liquid system between 5 and 8%, which should give rise to a linear shrinkage between 1.5 and 2%. In practice, when the linear contraction is measured, the result is only about 0.2–0.5% in processed acrylic, which is primarily attributed to the thermal contraction as the mould cools from the curing temperature.

The curing contraction is almost eliminated because the material is able to flow at the processing temperatures. Keeping the material under pressure after the curing reaction has finished allows the material to flow into any areas created by the curing contraction.

Gaseous porosity

This is volatilisation of the monomer. It is caused by the boiling of the monomer, particularly if too much has been added to the dough or if the temperature is raised too quickly, causing the exothermic curing reaction to generate temperature rises above the boiling point of the monomer (100.3°C). This potential problem can be eliminated by having a long curing period with a hold period at about 70°C, to allow the exothermic reaction within the processing flask to pass, before increasing the temperature for final processing (95°C).

Modern heat-cured acrylics are very flexible. If the correct powder/liquid ratio has been achieved the processing times can vary from 2 hours at 95°C (rapid cure) to 5 hours at 70°C and then 3 hours at 95°C (slow cure) without any observable differences in quality.

Processing strains

Restricting the dimensional change during cooling results in internal strains. Allowing them to relax would cause warpage, crazing or distortion. Cooling the flask slowly minimises the strains.

Relief of internal strains may cause crazing at the surface that has the appearance of a hazy or foggy area.

Flasking dentures

The flasking, packing and processing procedure for dentures is a relatively simple procedure, although technique-sensitive. There are several precautions that should be observed in order to achieve optimum results.

The procedure always results in an increase in vertical dimension of the denture. Consequently models should be articulated using a split-cast mounting technique in order that they may be remounted and the increase 'removed' post processing (see Figures 148–150).

The flasks must be in good condition in that they must close fully and accurately without resistance. If a flask fails to do this during the production of the two-part mould, air-blows, distortion or excess increase in vertical dimension may occur.

The coronal surfaces of the teeth must be free from wax to ensure that good adherence to the acrylic resin is achieved within the mould and to avoid tooth movement during processing.

Once the mould has been made, the wax needs to be removed without it soaking into the plaster. Failure to do this will prevent adequate isolation of the plaster and acrylic. Ideally, hot, non-recirculating water and a detergent or wax solvent should then be used to remove the softened wax.

When dry, but while still hot, all exposed surfaces of the plaster and stone mould should be painted with model separating medium. Ensure that this material does not 'puddle' around the teeth or coat the exposed denture teeth, thereby preventing good chemical bonding between teeth and acrylic resin.

The acrylic should be placed into the mould just before the dough reaches the 'snap dough' stage, to ensure that it will be forced into the surface details while under pressure. Note that the acrylic resin at the 'Snap dough' stage can be a little hard and may not fully press into all the detail within the mould and may also prevent the flasks being closed together properly.

The flasks should be closed under slow, constant pressure (80 psi) to allow the material to flow into the fine detail and the excess out of the mould.

The manufacturer's curing cycle should be observed to prevent curing contraction and gaseous porosity.

After processing a copper headed hammer should be used to open the flasks to avoid excessive force and prevent shock wave forces passing through the flask, plaster/stone block and denture, which could lead to the denture cracking because of excessive stress concentrations.

Techniques that help during the flasking procedure

Class IV die stone

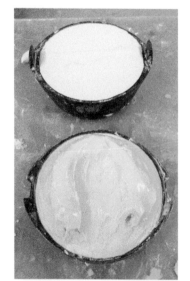

Figure 299

The use of vacuum mixed die stone in a thin layer over the entire wax denture improves the procedure in two ways. First, there is little risk of air blows in the surface of the mould, and secondly a weaker material may be used to form the bulk of mould, making de-flasking easier and with less risk of causing damage to the denture. Figure 299 shows Class IV die stone being used to create a hard but thin shell around the denture teeth and wax work during flasking. This is then backed with plaster of Paris, which makes de-flasking easier.

Silicone wafer

Heavy-bodied silicone may also be used to form the initial surface of the mould. Here care must be taken to ensure the material is rigid enough so that it does not distort under load. This is achieved by selecting a stiff, heavy-bodied silicone used in thin section with dental stone over the top to support it. Figure 300 shows silicone putty used to cover the teeth and wax work during flasking. This makes de-flasking much easier and safer and leads to a much cleaner denture. Staining can also still be carried out using this method.

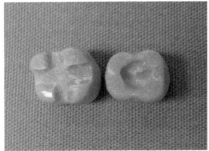

Figure 300

Bonding to artificial teeth

Bonding to acrylic teeth is aided significantly by grinding the surface of the teeth, complete wax removal prior to packing, and avoiding contamination with sodium alginate solution. Particular care must be taken when using composite teeth, as the retention can be poor. As a precaution, the teeth should be roughened or retention holes/grooves prepared as shown in Figure 301.

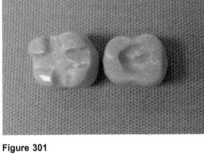

Figure 301

Porcelain teeth are presented with metal pins or diatoric holes to allow mechanical retention to the acrylic. Care should be taken to ensure that grinding during the placement of these teeth does not impair the integrity of these structures.

Injection moulding

Injection moulding has become relatively popular in the processing of PMMA. The main advantage is that the flask is closed tightly prior to the material being injected. This avoids the increase in vertical dimension that results from packing a two-part mould in the conventional manner.

Also of significance is the pressurised reservoir of material that remains attached to the mould throughout the curing process. This provides additional material to compensate for any contraction of the acrylic and keeps the acrylic resin under constant pressure during processing. Figure 302 shows an injection-moulding flask ready to place in the processing bath.

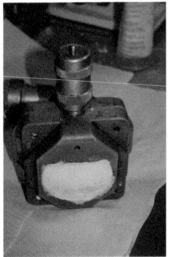

Figure 302

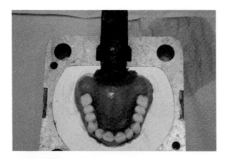

Figure 303

The procedure of flasking is similar to the conventional method with the exception that a wax sprue and dummy injection nozzle must be added to the distal border of the denture prior to topping the mould. The model is invested into one half of the flask, wax is then used, as shown in Figure 303, to link the denture base to the dummy injection nozzle used during investing. After boiling out the wax, the mould is re-assembled with the injection nozzle located in the flask. Figure 304a shows the invested denture with the wax removed and flasks open, Figure 304b shows the injection nozzle in place and in Figure 304c the two halves of the flask are secured together ready for PMMA injection.

Figure 305 shows the acrylic mix loaded into a dispenser. The mould and dispenser are then loaded into a pneumatic press that applies a constant load to the reservoir of acrylic, as shown in Figure 306.

After the mould is completely filled and no more movement of resin is observed, the dispenser and its protective shield can be removed (Figure 307a). A sprung cap is then screwed onto the end of the injection nozzle to maintain a constant pressure on the PMMA during processing (Figure 307b). This negates the need to place the flask into any kind of sprung clamp during processing.

After processing the sprung cap and injection nozzle are removed (Figure 308) and the denture de-vested as normal.

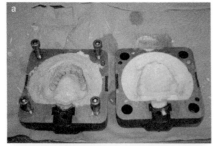
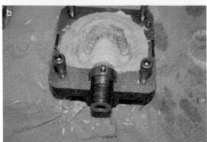
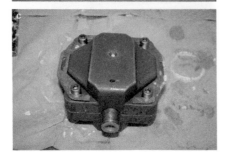

Figure 304

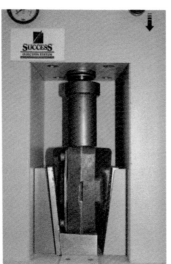

Figure 306

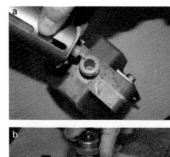
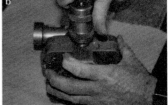

Figure 307

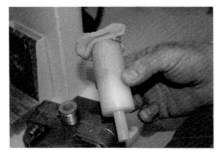

Figure 305

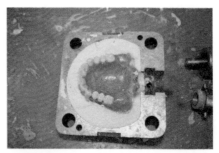

Figure 308

Gingival staining techniques

Staining of the labial surfaces of dentures is a relatively simple procedure to carry out, although practice is required to achieve predictable results. Characterising the dentures in this way is of particular benefit where high lip lines result in the acrylic being visible. In conjunction with gingival contouring and stippling, the results can be excellent. In Figure 309 various manufacturer's stain kits have been used to stain the maxillary and mandibular dentures but have produced nearly identical results. Stippling also helps to diffuse light entering the mouth and produce a more natural appearance.

Two examples of staining kits which are typical of the types available are described below. Both these techniques require practice in order to obtain reliable results.

The Candulor kit

The Candulor kit (Candulor AG, CH-8602 Wangen/ZH, Punten 4, Switzerland), of which there are heat and cold cure versions, contains three premixed colours and a range of intensive colours and veining fibres (Figure 310). The procedure for use is as follows.

1. The flasks are boiled out and isolated as normal and left to cool.

2. If using heat-curing acrylic, the base material is mixed and left to form dough as normal. If using cold-curing acrylic the base material is mixed after the staining procedure.

3. The coloured acrylic is mixed with a monomer that allows extended working time.

4. The instructions contain some examples of where to place the different coloured acrylic but generally these extend from light to dark, from cervical margin to labial sulcus. A typical 'map' of how stains should be applied is shown in Figure 311. Light is applied near the necks of the teeth then getting progressively darker towards the sulcus.

5. The acrylics are placed and should be layered over each other as shown in Figure 312 so they show a gradual transition between the colours and do not end up looking like a stick of rock!

6. The denture base resin is then packed behind the staining and the mould closed and processed as normal.

Care should be taken on polishing to ensure that the detail is not lost.

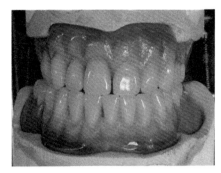

Figure 309

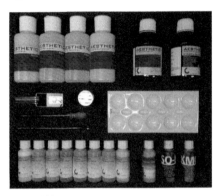

Figure 310

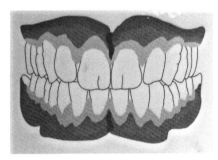

Figure 311

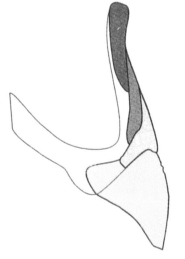

Figure 312

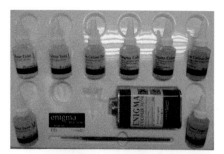

Figure 313

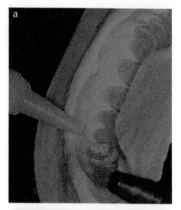

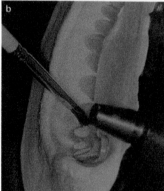

Figure 314

Schottlander

Schottlander (Davis Schottlander & Davis Ltd, Letchworth, Herts SG6 2WD, UK) produce a denture base stain system called the Enigma Colour Tone staining kit (Figure 313). This is used in a similar manner to the Candulor kit, but the coloured acrylic monomer and polymer are applied using a 'salt and vinegar' technique. The powder is placed into position within the mould and then 'wetted' with the monomer as shown in Figure 314. This is continued until the desired effect is achieved.

The denture base resin is then packed behind the staining and the mould closed and processed as normal.

Again, care should be taken on polishing to ensure that the detail is not lost.

Chapter 10 | FINISHING DENTURES

The processed dentures should be removed from the moulds using a saw or plaster cutters; however, the dentures should not be removed from the models at this stage.

After cleaning the dentures and model bases under running water, imperfections on the model base and articulating bases should be removed to ensure accurate fitting between the models and the articulator mounting plaster bases. The models can be re-secured back into these bases using a small amount of 'super glue' or by running molten sticky wax along the model/mounting plaster junction as shown in Figure 315.

Initially the centric locks should be engaged and the inter-cuspal position (ICP) contacts checked as shown in Figure 316. Note the incisal guidance pin is off the table, showing an increase in vertical dimension due to the 'flash' layer caused during processing in two-part flasks.

Grinding the premature occlusal contacts seen should reduce observed increases in vertical dimension. Note that fossae and cusp angles should be removed in preference to cusp tips to preserve the morphology of the teeth. To make adjustments, use articulating paper or cloth to highlight the contact as shown in Figure 317. The aim is to achieve occlusal contacts between cusp tip and fossae or marginal ridges (Figure 318).

Adjustments to premature contacts should continue until the increased vertical dimension is reduced and the incisal guidance pin touches the table (Figure 319) and until all cusp tips contact opposing fossae/marginal ridges.

For natural/conventional occlusions, contacts should be established between the palatal cusp of the upper tooth and the central fossa of the lower tooth as well as contact between the buccal cusp of the lower teeth and the central fossa of the upper teeth.

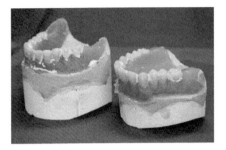

Figure 315

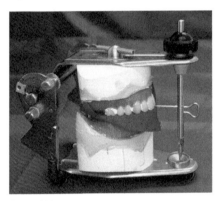

Figure 316

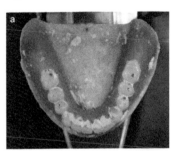

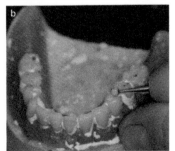

Figure 317

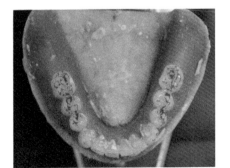

Figure 318

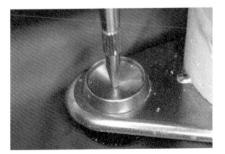

Figure 319

Techniques in Complete Denture Technology, First Edition. Tony Johnson, Duncan J. Wood.
© 2012 Tony Johnson and Duncan J. Wood. Published 2012 by Blackwell Publishing Ltd.

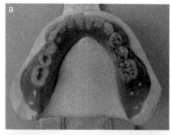

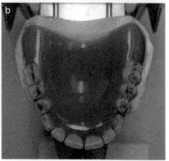

Figure 320

For lingualised occlusion, the contacts occur between the palatal cusp of the upper teeth and the central fossae of the lower teeth. The first premolars are different in that the contact is between the lower buccal cusp and upper central fossae.

These differences between natural and lingualised occlusion centric contacts are shown in Figure 320. The lingualised contacts (on the left side of both photographs as you look at them) shows the contacts are concentrated more over the centre of the ridges and are far fewer than the natural occlusion contacts.

Once centric contacts have been optimised the centric locks can be released and the lateral and protrusive excursions adjusted using a differently coloured articulating paper or cloth to differentiate between the centric and lateral contacts. The centric contacts should not be ground any further. As shown in Figure 321, premature contacts should be ground until a smooth excursion is seen, the incisal guidance pin stays on the table during the excursion and as many contacts as possible are maintained on both the working and balancing sides. Only the buccal upper and lingual lower contacts are ground; this is called the BULL rule and is established to preserve balancing contacts.

In lateral excursions the working side should have simultaneous contact between each tooth. This contact should be harmonious with the incisal pin on the incisal table as shown in Figure 322.

The balancing side should have at least one contact between the upper palatal cusp and lower buccal cusp as shown in Figure 323. In protrusion there should be a posterior contact to prevent tipping of the denture as shown in Figure 324. Protrusive excursions should see as many contacts as possible on both sides of the arch.

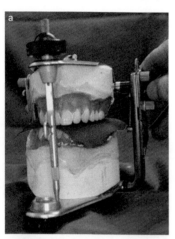

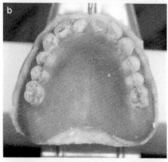

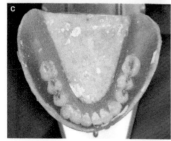

Figure 321

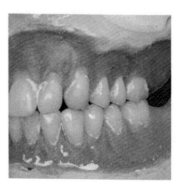

Figure 322

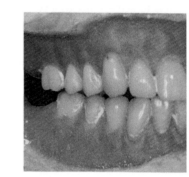

Figure 323

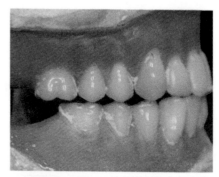

Figure 324

Similarly when adjusting contacts in the protrusive excursion, look for contacts on mesial facing slopes of lower teeth and distal facing slopes of upper teeth as shown in Figure 325.

Fine-tuning can be carried out using fine grinding-in paste. Place the paste between the teeth and while applying firm pressure to the upper arm of the articulator and run the teeth through each excursion and finally in circular motions, to simulate masticatory action and to remove any small interferences (Figure 326).

The dentures may now be removed from the models. This often breaks the alveolar ridge from the models, however the models should still support the dentures adequately if any check record procedures are necessary. (If large undercuts are present on the models it is better to grind away the model from inside the denture rather than risk cracking the denture by levering the denture off the model.)

Trim the dentures, taking care to preserve any detail that has been sculpted into the outer surfaces. Then polish using pumice and Tripoli polishing compound.

Where fine surface contouring, stippling or staining has been incorporated, a polishing paste should be used with goat hair brush to ensure the detail is not lost. Stippling may be carried out prior to polishing using a stippling bur. Figure 327 shows a stippling bur being used to texture the labial surface of the denture to diffuse light and create a more natural appearance.

Applying liquid paraffin to the surface to simulate its appearance after polishing may aid in assessing the effect of the stippling bur. Figure 328 shows liquid paraffin applied to the denture surface during stippling, simulating the effect likely to be seen when the dentures are in situ and covered in saliva. Note this demonstration denture has one side waxed up to look elderly and one side to look younger.

As shown in Figure 329, the fitting surface of the dentures should always be checked under magnification for any processing 'blips' or other sharp projections before sending to the clinic.

The dentures should be sterilised by immersing for 10 minutes in Perform sterilisation solution and stored in water for 24 hours prior to fitting to ensure that the relatively porous denture base is saturated in clean water rather than the first cup of coffee or red wine the patient drinks!

On fitting dentures, the extension and stability of the dentures should be checked, and the occlusion checked for any interferences. Small interferences should not be adjusted at this stage as the denture mucosa needs to adapt to the new denture base.

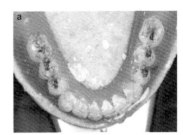

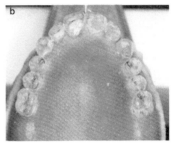

Figure 325

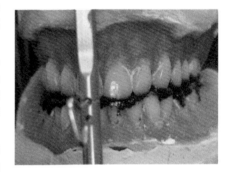

Figure 326

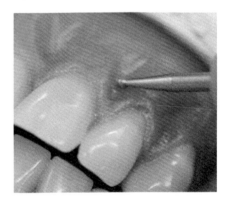

Figure 327

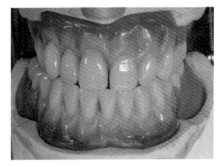

Figure 328

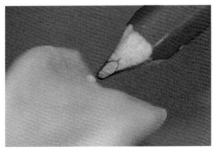

Figure 329

If, after one week, at the review stage, occlusal interferences are still present, then a 'check record' procedure should be carried out. This necessitates the dentures being 're-registered' and the lower model remounted on the articulator to the new registration. Occlusal grinding is then carried out again, as previously described, to achieve balanced occlusion and remove the occlusal interferences.

If gross occlusal interferences and obvious mistakes with the occlusion are seen at the fit stage a check record should be carried out immediately.

Chapter 11 | SPECIAL TECHNIQUES

Neutral zone dentures

Neutral zone dentures can be used for patients who have experienced difficulty wearing or functioning with their complete dentures. The technique involves shaping the 'polished' surfaces of the dentures to conform to the muscular actions of the lips, cheeks and tongue. This involves taking an impression of these muscles in their most activated positions using easily manipulated impression materials. The technique is usually used more with the lower denture than the upper denture.

A neutral zone denture technique is described below.

Clinical procedure

1. Construct the primary and secondary impressions, special trays and primary and working models as usual.

2. Construct the occlusal record blocks as usual. Construct an extra base as shown in Figure 330 with metal retention loops made of soft nickel silver wire, 1.25 mm diameter, to hold the neutral zone impression.

3. Carry out the occlusal registration as usual.

4. Use the extra base with the retention loops to record the neutral zone using a fluid impression material.

5. Check to ensure that the retention loops does not interfere with the musculature during functional movements; adjustments can easily be made using pliers.

6. Having checked the base for stability, load impression plaster, or a similarly fluid impression material, onto the base. The forming of the neutral zone impression is then carried out.

7. Before the neutral zone impression material sets, instruct the patient to make a series of functional movements of the lips, cheeks and tongue. Exaggeratedly saying the letters 'E' (Figure 331a) and 'O' (Figure 331b) and trying to touch the nose with the tip of the tongue, can produce these functional movements.

The placement of too much impression material onto the base will not cause problems. Excess material can easily be displaced upwards into the 'upper' denture space where it can be removed with a sharp knife.

If insufficient material is loaded onto the base, the material of choice should allow for additions to be made and the procedure repeated.

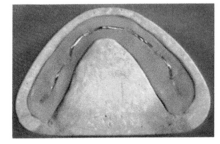

Figure 330

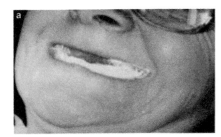

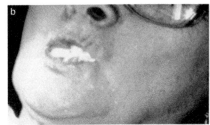

Figure 331

Techniques in Complete Denture Technology, First Edition. Tony Johnson, Duncan J. Wood.
© 2012 Tony Johnson and Duncan J. Wood. Published 2012 by Blackwell Publishing Ltd.

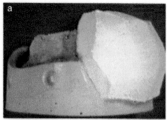
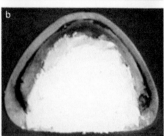
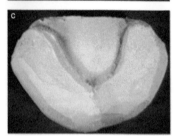

Figure 332

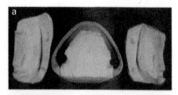
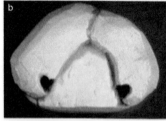
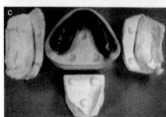

Figure 333

The final impression should be perfectly stable in situ, the impression representing the patient's functional denture space.

Technical procedure

1. Mount the secondary models and occlusal registration blocks into an articulator.

2. Remove the lower block and replace it with the impression of the neutral zone/denture space. Construct a three-part sectional overcast around the impression and the model using dental plaster as shown in Figure 332a–c.

3. Remove the wax rim from the lower occlusal registration block. Place the base back onto the lower model and re-assemble the three-part sectional overcast around the lower model (Figure 333a,b).

4. Pour molten wax through the two holes prepared in the overcasts in the retro-molar pad region onto the lower base until the mould is full to create an exact wax replica of the patient's neutral zone/denture space (Figure 333c).

5. Adjust any discrepancies in the height of the 'new lower block' on the articulator, against the upper occlusal registration block.

6. Set up the upper teeth as normal.

7. Set up the lower teeth to the uppers, using the plaster overcast as a guide to ensure that the lower teeth do not encroach beyond the recorded neutral zone/denture space. This may necessitate the reduction of the bucco-lingual width of the lower posterior teeth and the cingula of the lower anterior teeth Figure 334a,b.

8. Perform a try-in of the waxed-up dentures. Make the usual checks, paying special attention to the muscular action upon the lower denture. Remove any overextension of the 'polished' surface of the denture (this is particularly evident in the lingual shelf area). The lower denture should be stable and comfortable during function and speech.

9. Finish and fit the dentures using normal techniques.

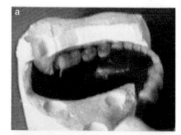
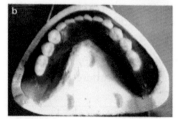

Figure 334

A simpler partial neutral zone denture technique, only involving the lower anterior teeth region, is shown in Figure 335. This is carried out at the registration stage using the registration rim to hold the impression of the anterior section of the neutral zone. It is quicker and does not require a separate base.

Implant-retained complete dentures

Implant-retained dentures fall into two main categories:

- patient-removable implant-retained dentures, which are usually retained on no more than two implants using either a stud (Figure 336a,b) or bar type (Figure 336c,d) attachment; and
- fixed implant-retained dentures, which are permanently screwed directly to usually four or more implants and obtain no support from the underlying tissues.

Figure 337a shows a fixed, cast gold beam, PMMA maxillary denture retained by six implants. Figure 337b shows a computer-designed, computer-milled (CAD/CAM) cobalt chromium framework onto which a PMMA denture will be constructed. Figure 337c shows a cast gold framework with a PMMA denture processed around it. Note that although the PMMA denture base is in need of replacement due to wear, the cast gold framework is still perfect.

Fixed implant-retained dentures cannot really be classed as dentures as they do not usually gain any support from the alveolar or soft tissues and are not patient removable. Patient-removable dentures, other the other hand, although they have two implants for retention, should be treated exactly the same as conventional complete dentures as they will gain most of their support from the underlying tissues, the implants mainly aiding with retention not support! Mucocompressive impressions, which are functionally extended, are essential to obtain good stability (remember that the two implants are usually in the canine region of the mouth and do not afford support for the posterior part of the denture).

The attachments chosen to work in conjunction with implants in these cases should ideally be resilient not rigid ones. This will allow the denture to 'sink into the mucosa' without putting an undue strain onto the implants or through the denture base during function.

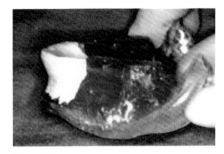

Figure 335

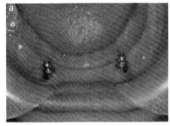

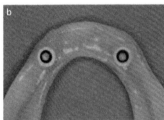

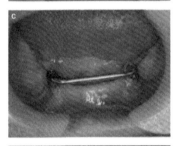

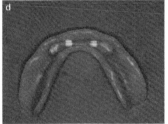

Figure 336

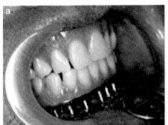
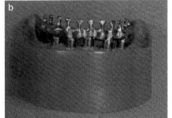
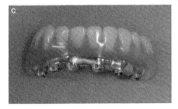

Figure 337

Index

Page numbers in italics denote figures; those in bold denote tables.